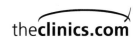

# CARDIOLOGY CLINICS

Adult Congenital Heart Disease

GUEST EDITOR
Gary D. Webb, MD

CONSULTING EDITOR
Michael H. Crawford, MD

November 2006 • Volume 24 • Number 4

**SAUNDERS**

An Imprint of Elsevier, Inc.
PHILADELPHIA   LONDON   TORONTO   MONTREAL   SYDNEY   TOKYO

**W.B. SAUNDERS COMPANY**
*A Division of Elsevier Inc.*

Elsevier Inc. • 1600 John F. Kennedy Blvd., Suite 1800 • Philadelphia, Pennsylvania 19103-2899

http://www.theclinics.com

**CARDIOLOGY CLINICS**
November 2006
Editor: Karen Sorensen

**Volume 24, Number 4**
**ISSN 0733-8651**
**ISBN 1-4160-3877-9**

Reprints. For copies of 100 or more, of articles in this publication, please contact the Commercial Reprints Department, Elsevier Inc., 360 Park Avenue South, New York, New York 10010-1710. Tel. (212) 633-3813 Fax: (212) 462-1935 email: reprints@elsevier.com.

The ideas and opinions expressed in *Cardiology Clinics* do not necessarily reflect those of the Publisher. The Publisher does not assume any responsibility for any injury and/or damage to persons or property arising out of or related to any use of the material contained in this periodical. The reader is advised to check the appropriate medical literature and the product information currently provided by the manufacturer of each drug to be administered to verify the dosage, the method and duration of administration, or contraindications. It is the responsibility of the treating physician or other health care professional, relying on independent experience and knowledge of the patient, to determine drug dosages and the best treatment for the patient. Mention of any product in this issue should not be construed as endorsement by the contributors, editors, or the Publisher of the product or manufacturers' claims.

*Cardiology Clinics* (ISSN 0733-8651) is published quarterly by Elsevier Inc., 360 Park Avenue South, New York, NY 10010-1710. Months of issue are February, May, August, and November. Business and editorial Offices: 1600 John F. Kennedy Blvd., Suite 1800, Philadelphia, PA 19103-2899. Customer Service Office: 6277 Sea Harbor Drive, Orlando, FL 32887-4800. Periodicals postage paid at New York, NY, and additional mailing offices. Subscription prices are $198.00 per year for US individuals, $302.00 per year for US institutions, $99.00 per year for US students and residents, $242.00 per year for Canadian individuals, $367.00 per year for Canadian institutions, $264.00 per year for international individuals, $367.00 per year for international institutions and $132.00 per year for Canadian and foreign students/residents. To receive student/resident rate, orders must be accompanied by name of affiliated institution, data of term, and the *signature* of program/residency coordinator on institution letterhead. Orders will be billed at individual rate until proof of status is received. Foreign air speed delivery is included in all *Clinics* subscription prices. All prices are subject to change without notice. POSTMASTER: Send address changes to *Cardiology Clinics*, Elsevier Periodicals Customer Service, 6277 Sea Harbor Drive, Orlando, FL 32887-4800. **Customer Service: 1-800-654-2452 (US). From outside of the US, call 1-407-345-1000.**

*Cardiology Clinics* is also published in Spanish by McGraw-Hill Interamericana Editores S. A., P.O. Box 5-237, 06500, Mexico D. F., Mexico; in Portuguese by Reichmann and Alfonso Editores Rio de Janeiro, Brazil; and in Greek by Dimitrios P. Lagos, 8 Pondon Street, GR115-28 Ilissia, Greece.

*Cardiology Clinics* is covered in *Index Medicus, Excerpta Medica, The Cumulative Index to Nursing and Allied Health Literature* (INAHL).

Printed in the United States of America.

# CONSULTING EDITOR

**MICHAEL H. CRAWFORD, MD,** Professor of Medicine, Lucie Stern Chair in Cardiology, University of California San Francisco; and Chief of Clinical Cardiology, University of California, San Francisco Medical Center, San Francisco, California

# GUEST EDITOR

**GARY D. WEBB, MD,** Director, Philadelphia Adult Congenital Heart Center, Children's Hospital of Philadelphia, and the Hospital of the University of Pennsylvania, Philadelphia, Pennsylvania

# CONTRIBUTORS

**LEE BENSON, MD, FRCP(C),** Director, Cardiac Diagnostic and Interventional Unit, Division of Cardiology, Hospital for Sick Children, Toronto, Ontario, Canada

**FRANCOIS P. BERNIER, MD,** Assistant Professor, Department of Medical Genetics, University of Calgary, Calgary, Alberta; and Director, Clinical Genetics Unit, Calgary Health Region, Alberta, Canada

**GERHARD-PAUL DILLER, MD,** Adult Congenital Heart Centre and Centre for Pulmonary Hypertension, Royal Brompton Hospital and National Heart & Lung Institute, Imperial College, London, United Kingdom

**KONSTANTINOS DIMOPOULOS, MD,** Adult Congenital Heart Centre and Centre for Pulmonary Hypertension, Royal Brompton Hospital and National Heart & Lung Institute, Imperial College, London, United Kingdom

**MICHAEL A. GATZOULIS, MD, PhD, FACC,** Professor of Cardiology and Director, Adult Congenital Heart Disease Centre, Royal Brompton and Harefield NHS Trust and the National Heart and Lung Institute at Imperial College, London, United Kingdom

**JANE HEGGIE, MD, FRCP,** Assistant Professor of Anesthesia, Toronto General Hospital, Toronto, Ontario, Canada

**ERIC HORLICK, MD, FRCP(C),** University Health Network, Toronto, Ontario, Canada

**MARK R. JOHNSON, PhD, MRCP, MRCOG,** Consultant Obstetrician and Honorary Senior Lecturer, Academic Obstetrics and Gynaecology, Chelsea and Westminster Hospital and Imperial College, London, United Kingdom

**HENRYK KAFKA, MD, FRCPC, FACC,** Visiting Consultant Cardiologist and Honorary Senior Lecturer, Adult Congenital Heart Disease Centre, Royal Brompton and Harefield NHS Trust and the National Heart and Lung Institute at Imperial College, London, United Kingdom; and Division of Cardiology, Queen's University, Kingston, Ontario, Canada

**JACEK KARSKI, MD, FRCP,** Associate Professor of Anesthesia and Director of Cardiovascular Anesthesia and Intensive Care, Toronto General Hospital, University Health Network, University of Toronto, Toronto, Ontario, Canada

**ALISON KNAUTH, MD, PhD,** Boston Adult Congenital Heart Program, Boston; Children's Hospital Boston, Boston; Brigham and Women's Hospital, Boston; and Harvard Medical School, Boston, Massachusetts

**ADRIENNE H. KOVACS, PhD,** Cardiac Psychology, Division of Cardiology, University Health Network, Toronto, Ontario, Canada

**PETER MCLAUGHLIN, MD, FRCP(C),** Peterborough Regional Health Centre, Peterborough, Ontario, Canada

**DISTY PEARSON, PA-C,** Physician Assistant, Boston Adult Congenital Heart (BACH) Service, Department of Cardiology, Brigham and Women's Hospital, Beth Israel Deaconess Medical Center, and Children's Hospital, Boston, Massachusetts

**MASSIMO F. PIEPOLI, MD, PhD,** Department of Clinical Cardiology, National Heart and Lung Institute, Imperial College, London, United Kingdom; and Heart Failure Unit, Cardiac Department, G. Da Saliceto Polichirugico Hospital, Piacenza, Italy

**ANDREW N. REDINGTON, MD,** Head of Cardiology, Hospital for Sick Children, Toronto, Canada

**JOHN REISS, PhD,** Institute for Child Health Policy, University of Florida, Gainesville, Florida

**ARWA SAIDI, MB, BCh, FACC,** Associate Professor, Departments of Pediatrics and Internal Medicine, University of Florida, Gainesville, Florida

**SAMUEL F. SEARS, PhD,** Associate Professor, Department of Clinical and Health Psychology, College of Public Health and Health Professions, University of Florida, Gainesville, Florida

**CANDICE SILVERSIDES, MD,** Assistant Professor of Medicine, Division of Cardiology, University Health Network, University of Toronto, Toronto General Hospital, Toronto, Ontario, Canada

**RENEE SPAETGENS, MD,** Resident, Department of Medical Genetics, University of Calgary, Calgary, Alberta, Canada

**AMY VERSTAPPEN, MEd,** President, Adult Congenital Heart Association, Philadelphia, Pennsylvania

**GARY D. WEBB, MD,** Director, Philadelphia Adult Congenital Heart Center, Children's Hospital of Philadelphia, and the Hospital of the University of Pennsylvania, Philadelphia, Pennsylvania

# CONTENTS

cardiac development and to determine the impact of mutations in these genes in the pathogenesis of syndromic and nonsyndromic congenital heart defects. Some of these advances in genetic knowledge are being translated into clinical care, raising the question of what role this knowledge should have in the adult congenital heart disease (ACHD) clinic. The authors summarize the clinical and molecular advances relevant to the care and genetic counseling of ACHD patients and explore the role of genetic care providers in an ACHD clinic.

Anesthesia for adults with congenital heart disease has many challenging physiologic considerations. Collaborative relationships of a multidisciplinary team including cardiology, cardiac surgery, anesthesiology, and intensive care are essential to ensure positive outcomes in this population for noncardiac and cardiac surgery.

The successful pediatric management of congenital heart disease has resulted in increasing numbers of these patients in the reproductive age group and increasing clinical challenges for their physicians. These challenges can be met successfully, with improved results for mother and child, through a concerted comprehensive team approach that relies on a thorough understanding of the patient's underlying cardiac pathology and its anticipated interaction with the pregnancy, and ongoing close evaluation and communication with a team of trained and experienced specialists, including (but not limited to) cardiologists, obstetricians, anesthetists, pediatricians, clinical nurse specialists, and clinical geneticists. Such teams are not always available locally and it will be necessary to refer medium- and high-risk patients to a specialized tertiary care center.

In addition to monitoring and treating the cardiac disease, patients benefit from health professionals recognizing and managing the potential psychosocial consequences of growing up with congenital heart disease. Working groups from Europe and North America have emphasized the benefit of inclusion of specialized mental health care for adult congenital heart disease (ACHD) patients. This article reviews the evidence that ACHD patients have special and unique psychosocial needs and outlines ways in which psychologists can be integrated into multidisciplinary ACHD care teams. There are three professional domains in which clinical health psychologists can contribute to an ACHD team: provision of clinical services, multidisciplinary research, and professional education. Considerations for incorporating psychology into ACHD teams are also presented.

This article focuses on the process of transition and transfer of care of young adults with complex congenital heart disease. It defines the transition process and briefly discusses its history. It reviews the important aspects of transition, outlines the key elements of a successful transition program, and provides a curriculum appropriate for the young adult with congenital heart disease. Finally, it identifies the barriers to transfer of care, discusses the importance of a policy on timing, outlines the components of adult provider services that may be needed, and reviews the steps to an orderly transfer process.

# FORTHCOMING ISSUES

# RECENT ISSUES

---

## VISIT OUR WEB SITE

The Clinics are now available online!
**Access your subscription at www.theclinics.com**

ELSEVIER
SAUNDERS

Cardiol Clin 24 (2006) ix

CARDIOLOGY
CLINICS

# Foreword

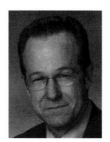

Michael H. Crawford, MD
*Consulting Editor*

Dr. Webb has organized a unique issue on the adult with congenital heart disease (CHD). Dr. Webb runs a multidisciplinary CHD unit in Philadelphia that is a model for other such units. Thus, I was delighted that he had agreed to guest edit this issue. His unique perspective is evident in the first article, which presents the patient's perspective on the care of adults with CHD. Although this may seem strange, patient involvement is a critical part of most adult CHD units. Our unit at University of California, San Francisco and the one at Stanford University recently held a continuing medical education conference on adult CHD and invited our patients. More patients showed up than caregivers.

Much of this issue explores the concept of the multidisciplinary approach that these patients require. There are articles on anesthesia, surgical, interventional, genetic, obstetric, and psychological issues surrounding the care of these patients. One major issue covered is the orderly transition from pediatric to adult cardiologist. In my experience, this is one of the more contentious issues with these patients. There is an understandable tendency for pediatric cardiologists to hold onto these patients well into adulthood, which in some circumstances, is in the patient's best interest. On the other hand, many adult cardiologists believe that pediatric patients should be transferred to them at the first signs of puberty. This also can

make sense because of the new risks of venereal disease, pregnancy, drug abuse, and so forth, that adolescence brings.

Finally, the last articles are on two important topics. Tetralogy of Fallot is the most common cyanotic heart disease and is usually repaired in early childhood. Currently, post repair pulmonic regurgitation is a major issue that is fully discussed by Redington. Besides survival, the other major goal of care in CHD patients is their ability to lead normal lives. The latter requires an ability to be active. Thus, the last article, on exercise capacity in CHD patients, is very topical.

I believe that the readers will agree that this is an outstanding issue by noted experts in the field from both sides of the Atlantic that will provide those caring for adult CHD patients with considerable practical knowledge and that will help them organize their own adult CHD units.

Michael H. Crawford, MD
*Division of Cardiology*
*Department of Medicine*
*University of California*
*San Francisco Medical Center*
*505 Parnassus Avenue, Box 0124*
*San Francisco, CA 94143-0124, USA*

*E-mail address:* crawfordm@medicine.ucsf.edu

CARDIOLOGY
CLINICS

Cardiol Clin 24 (2006) xi–xii

# Preface

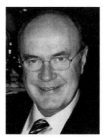

Gary D. Webb, MD
*Guest Editor*

This issue of *Cardiology Clinics* is devoted to the growing field of adult congenital heart disease (ACHD). The central roles of cardiologists, cardiovascular surgeons, and nurses are well understood. In recent years in the United States, there has been a major growth in the number of centers caring for adult patients with congenital heart defects. There are now approximately 60 ACHD centers in the United States, many of which have just started up in the past few years. What role should these centers play in the care of ACHD patients?

The first article offers an important and unique perspective, that of the ACHD patient. The lead author is Amy Verstappen, president of the Adult Congenital Heart Association, an important ACHD advocacy organization. For the first time in the medical literature, she and her colleagues articulate the perspectives of the ACHD patient. Issues discussed include the impact of overly pessimistic and overly optimistic prognoses, common patient misperceptions and knowledge gaps, frustrations and dangerous encounters in the medical system, and living with invisible disabilities.

One of the implications of establishing an ACHD clinic is that these patients, many of whom have quite complex anatomy and physiology, require multidisciplinary care. How does an ACHD center develop multidisciplinary capability? What are the elements of multidisciplinary care that need to be considered? What can consultants and team members be expected to contribute to the care of these patients?

The second article defines the role of cardiac catheterization in a modern ACHD facility. The authors discuss the planning of the procedure, the potential pitfalls to be anticipated, and the equipment needed for the procedure. They then discuss the performance of the cardiac catheterization. They go on to outline the current role of heart catheterization in the era of advanced noninvasive imaging, with a focus on interventional procedures. Finally, the authors look at new and emerging interventions and speculate on the future of diagnostic heart catheterization in the ACHD patient.

The next multidisciplinary topic considers the role of the geneticist in an ACHD center, summarizing the clinical and molecular advances relevant to the care and genetic counseling of ACHD patients and exploring the role of genetic care providers in such clinics.

Although the key role of the cardiovascular surgeon is well understood, we are reminded that a strong surgical program requires a multidisciplinary team of its own. The next articles focus on the role of the anesthesiologist in caring for ACHD patients. The authors review the preoperative assessment of the ACHD patient; the pharmacology of anesthetic agents; and the

doi:10.1016/j.ccl.2006.09.002

anesthesiologist's role in noncardiac surgical procedures, diagnostic and interventional procedures,
and congenital heart surgery on adult patients.

ACHD patients are relatively young, so the
management of the pregnant patient is an important part of ACHD patient care. The group from
the Royal Brompton Hospital describes their
model for meeting this challenge using a comprehensive team approach that includes evaluation
and communication with a team of trained and
experienced specialists, including cardiologists,
obstetricians, anesthetists, pediatricians, clinical
nurse specialists, and clinical geneticists.

The next article focuses on the role of the
psychologist in ACHD patients. The authors
remind us that patients benefit from having their
caregivers recognize and manage the potential
psychosocial consequences of growing up with
congenital heart disease. The role of the psychologist integrated into multidisciplinary ACHD care
teams is reviewed in relation to the provision of
clinical services, multidisciplinary research, and
professional education.

The transition process prepares children and
adolescents with congenital heart defects to learn
how to manage their own health care as they enter
adult life. The transfer of adolescent patients to
adult care facilities should follow such a transition
process wherever competent adult care is available. The next article focuses on these issues. It
outlines the key elements of a successful transition
program, and provides a general curriculum
appropriate for the young adult with congenital
heart disease. It also identifies barriers to the
transfer of care, discusses the importance of
a policy on the timing of transfer, and reviews
the steps to an orderly transfer process.

The last two articles depart from the prevailing
theme. The first deals with the critically important
issue of pulmonary regurgitation in patients who
have had repairs of tetralogy of Fallot. Andrew
Redington takes a fresh and critical look at this
very important topic. He describes the primary
determinants of pulmonary regurgitation, the
methods by which pulmonary regurgitation is
measured, and some of the pitfalls in the assessment of this condition. He points out that
although our ability to measure pulmonary incompetence has improved significantly, there remain important pitfalls to its assessment in the
individual patient, and that our understanding of
its implications remains rather unsophisticated.

The final article represents a unique and
important synthesis of our knowledge about
exercise intolerance in ACHD patients. The authors discuss the assessment of exercise intolerance, the mechanisms of reduced exercise
capacity, neurohormonal activation, the prognostic value of parameters of exercise intolerance,
and the means of improving the exercise capacity
of ACHD patients.

It has been a pleasure for me to have worked
with these excellent colleagues to create an issue
presenting important and unique new perspectives
that can be used to improve the care of adult
patients with congenital heart defects. We anticipate considerable progress in the next decade,
and hope that the information provided here will
help guide the growth and development of high-
quality ACHD programs.

Gary D. Webb, MD
*Philadelphia Adult Congenital Heart Center*
*6 Penn Tower*
*3400 Spruce Street*
*Philadelphia, PA 19104-4283, USA*

*E-mail address:* Gary.webb@uphs.upenn.edu

ELSEVIER
SAUNDERS

CARDIOLOGY
CLINICS

Cardiol Clin 24 (2006) 515–529

# Adult Congenital Heart Disease: the Patient's Perspective

Amy Verstappen, MEd[a],*, Disty Pearson, PA-C[b],
Adrienne H. Kovacs, PhD[c]

[a]Adult Congenital Heart Association, 6757 Greene Street, Philadelphia, PA 19119, USA
[b]Boston Adult Congenital Heart (BACH) Service, Brigham and Woman's Hospital,
Departments of Cardiology, 300 Longwood Avenue, Boston, MA 02115, USA
[c]Cardiac Psychology, Division of Cardiology, University Health Network,
399 Bathurst Street, 1-West-414, Toronto, ON M5T 2N2, Canada

In addressing the patient's perspective in congenital heart disease (CHD), we must first acknowledge that there are many patient perspectives. The wide variability in diagnoses, age at diagnosis, treatment, and outcomes that makes CHD medically complex also results in a highly heterogeneous patient population and set of life experiences. Although there have been attempts to correlate specific defects with specific psychosocial outcomes, patients born with the same anatomy can have widely varied experiences. For example, consider three 40-year-old patients who have atrial septal defects. One patient, surgically repaired as an infant, considers herself cured, has not seen a cardiologist in 35 years, and is asymptomatic. The second is newly diagnosed, having developed symptoms after the birth of her second child, and is now awaiting repair. The third, born in a rural area and not referred for closure, has experienced life-long disability, developed Eisenmenger's syndrome, and has limited treatment options. Although the underlying defect is the same, the experience and impact of this anatomy is profoundly different in each case.

Amid this broad diversity, however, certain patterns of experience and perspective emerge, and these are known to the Adult Congenital Heart Association (ACHA), the only adult congenital heart disease (ACHD) patient advocacy group in the United States. Although the existing educational, psychosocial, and quality-of-life research is referenced in this article, the primary focus is on patient reports, drawn primarily from ACHA participant experiences. ACHD literature contains little that is written by the patients themselves. When ACHD patients share experiences with each other, many of the issues and challenges identified fall outside of the existing published literature.

To illustrate these perspectives, the authors provide quotations drawn from the ACHA discussion board at the Web site achaheart.org, which currently has over 900 registered participants with over 14,000 posted discussion topics. The authors also draw from their own experiences working with the adult congenital heart community as ACHD health advocate and peer support leader, midlevel health professional, and psychologist; the lead author is also informed by her own experiences as a survivor of complex CHD. The authors recognize that this approach is largely subjective and anecdotal; however, by offering this alternate perspective in which the primary concerns identified by the patients are addressed, the authors hope to prompt new research and new solutions.

The primary goals of this article are (1) to provide readers with "patients'-eye views" of the challenges of living with CHD and (2) to suggest implications for health care professionals. In

---

* Corresponding author.
*E-mail address:* amyv@achaheart.org
(A. Verstappen).

selecting topics, the authors particularly focused on areas in which the gap between the patient and medical perspective is most likely to negatively impact health care delivery and patient well-being. The focus initially is on themes with a more medical focus, including the impact of being told one was "cured," the impact of growing up as a "miracle baby," medical misinformation among patients, and commonly reported frustrations when navigating the medical system. The authors also address concerns raised by living with an invisible disability and confronting new health challenges. In addition to these more medical themes, the question of normalcy and the ways in which CHD can be a "gift" are also addressed. The article concludes with a discussion of the importance of ACHD patient associations. Each section identifies recommended best practices for the health care providers, and these recommendations are summarized in Box 1.

## Issue 1: the myth of "the cure"

[Patient 1] In 1973, when I was 17 years old, my cardiologist ended my annual visit by saying, "I don't need to see you anymore." While I don't recall his exact words, the essence was, "We've seen you through adolescence. That was the worrisome part. Now go live your life."

[Patient 2] I had a follow-up cath when I was five years old and the doctors told my parents that the result of the surgery was excellent, so I was "fixed." The terms *total correction* and *fixed* were used frequently by the doctors and they were used both synonymously and interchangeably...I saw an adult cardiologist for an evaluation at puberty [and]...did not see a cardiologist for between twenty-five and thirty years...I had an EKG annually. When I started with my current primary care practitioner in 1996, he started doing echoes every two years to "monitor" my heart as I was getting older.... But, like everyone before him, he said that I was "fixed."

Denial, lack of compliance, transition difficulties, and lack of education about one's defect are barriers to care commonly referenced in the cardiac literature. An additional commonly reported reason for no longer seeing a cardiologist, however, is being explicitly graduated from cardiac care. Many complex patients, particularly those who underwent surgery before 1980, report being told that they no longer needed to see a cardiologist, and many adults who have CHD report believing themselves "cured" following childhood or adolescent surgeries.

---

## Box 1. Recommended best practices for interactions with adults who have congenital heart disease

*Practices to avoid*
- Using terms such as fixed, cured, or complete repair
- Withholding known negative information
- Making predictions unsupported by data (eg, "This is your last surgery," "You won't live to see thirty")
- Relying on patient reports of normal functional capacity without objective testing
- Asking patients to compare themselves to "normal people"
- Confusing quality of life with health status

*Practices to promote*
- Educating for life-long self-advocacy and self-care
- Sharing data or acknowledging lack of data
- Encouraging optimism and planning for the future
- Providing copies of medical records
- Assessing function through serial testing
- Soliciting and respecting the patient's point of view
- Providing mental health resources
- Providing access to peer support

---

These reports should not be surprising given the lack of knowledge about long-term ACHD outcomes at the time and the commonly held belief that these surgeries were curative. What is more surprising is that many adult patients report that the misperception that they are "fixed" has been reinforced rather than corrected by their current health providers. The 32nd Bethesda Conference ("Care of the Adult with Congenital Heart Disease") categorized cardiac defects as being of mild, moderate, or great complexity (Appendix 1) [1]. Patients of moderate and great complexity should receive regular care at a specialty adult congenital cardiology program. For the purposes of this article, the authors refer to patients who have defects of moderate and great complexity as "complex." When complex patients are cared for by primary care providers without being referred to even a community-level cardiologist, this lack of referral can itself provide further evidence to the patient that they are "cured."

Another issue that bears further examination is the terminology of many congenital cardiac surgeries. Adult patients often refer to phrases such as "complete surgical correction" or "total surgical repair" to explain their perception of being fixed. To those unfamiliar with the complexities of CHD, these phrases can imply that the heart is "totally corrected" (ie, cured). ACHA's current experience with the pediatric congenital heart community suggests that despite the extensive data on residua and sequelae in complex CHD now available [2–4], today's children may still be at risk from language-based misperception. For example, in ACHA encounters with survivors of the arterial switch for transposition of the great arteries, parent statements that the child now has "normal heart anatomy" because she or he underwent an "anatomic repair" are common; few understand that an arterial switch, like virtually all complex CHD surgery, leaves behind abnormal hemodynamics and anatomy [5]. Such phrases may also contribute to the general community provider's lack of awareness of ACHD as a chronic disease. Modifying the terminology in CHD surgeries might reduce the misperception of cure and more accurately reflect current knowledge of complex CHD. As indicated in Appendix 1, few surgeries are considered curative.

The possibility that many complex ACHD patients perceive themselves as graduates of cardiac care is supported by data suggesting that only a minority of adults living with CHD continue to seek appropriate levels of care. For example, in the Natural History Study, 40% of patients studied had not had a cardiac examination in over 10 years [6]. Similarly, a study from the Canadian Adult Congenital Heart Network Consortium reported that only 37% to 47% of patients had successfully transitioned from pediatric cardiology care to adult medicine; 27% had not been evaluated since turning 18 years old [7]. This rate of transition is expected to be lower in the United States given the more organized nature of the Canadian care system, the frequent transfer of patients to adult CHD clinics at age 18, and the lack of financial barriers to medical care. In 2005, 59 self-described American ACHD clinics responding to an ACHA/International Society for Adult Congenital Cardiac Disease (ISACCD) survey reported a combined ACHD patient population of fewer than

34,000 per year; this number is likely an overestimate given that patient numbers were self-reported, often estimated, and included patients treated at more than one center. This survey indicates that a very small percentage of the estimated 500,000 American complex ACHD patients are being treated at an ACHD clinic.

In addition, until a more representative sample of the patient population is available for study, the generalization of research conclusions is limited due to biases in sample selection. The experiences of the minority of ACHD patients followed in pediatric and specialized ACHD facilities might not reflect the entire ACHD patient population. For example, these patients may be more likely to have health issues than those who perceive themselves as fixed and have left cardiac care. Population-based studies are essential to developing an accurate understanding of the long-term outcomes in ACHD, and ACHA strongly endorses the development of a national ACHD registry.

*Implications for health care providers*

Individuals working with pediatric and adult patients must avoid misleading language and clearly communicate to patients and families that those who have CHD, by definition, do not have normal hearts and those who have more complex CHD need life-long specialized cardiac care. Individuals working with adult patients must also acknowledge the possibility that many adults who have complex CHD consider themselves graduated from cardiac care due to misinformation provided by past and present health care providers. This acknowledgment calls for different action than if one sees ACHD patients as "in denial" because denial implies that the patient understands on some level that she or he needs cardiac care. Providing the best possible care to congenital heart survivors demands reaching out beyond the existing patient base and working with patient groups and others to promote community outreach, patient identification, and education regarding appropriate referral. The emerging consensus in congenital heart care is that health surveillance matters; delays in care can result in needless disability and loss of life.

### Issue 2: "miracle babies" and "lost causes"

[Patient 1] When I was three months old, I was diagnosed. The doctors looked at my parents and said, "Take her home and love her, she won't live to be one."

For ACHD patients born in the era when congenital heart surgery was in its infancy, the experience of having been a "miracle baby," although rarely referenced in the ACHD literature, can also be prominent in many patients' self-identity. When ACHD patients meet, one common topic of conversation is sharing these early experiences. For many patients too young to remember these encounters when they occurred, these stories are not memories but rather retellings of frequently recounted family lore. These stories typically begin with the statement that the child was not expected to survive and then include the extraordinary efforts the family went through to gain their child access to what was then rare, difficult to access, and sometimes extremely risky surgery. Even patients born when interventions had become more routine are often able to recount the moment that their parents were told their child would not live without surgery. For those who experienced "complete repairs," these stories typically end with the miracle of their surgery and successful survival.

In contrast, ACHD patients ineligible for surgery or only "partially repaired" often report the opposite experience: on-going, explicit statements by medical professionals that they would not live long.

> [Patient 2] After my Mustard, the surgeon said I'd never live to see my fifth birthday. When I was diagnosed with CHF, I was given three years to live ("five, if you're lucky"). I was sixteen, and my pediatric cardiologist thought I wouldn't make it through my sophomore year in college. I didn't find out until years later that he called my mom that afternoon and apologized for not being able to save me.

Not surprisingly, these kinds of predictions can result in a fear of death and difficulty planning for the future. Decisions such as pursuing higher education, working toward a career, establishing savings, or even developing long-term relationships may be avoided if one does not anticipate living into adulthood. At the extreme, some adults who have CHD reported engaging in highly risky behavior such as illegal drug use because they believed they did not have a future to put at risk. When these individuals do not die as expected, they may struggle with the migration into an adulthood for which they did not prepare.

More surprisingly, many ACHD patients report that rather than bringing on feelings of despair or passivity, statements of expected non-survival functioned as a challenge to prove the experts wrong.

> [Patient 3] I adapted the "I'll show them" attitude. I can do whatever I want no matter what anyone else tells me because the only person who limits me is me. So I celebrate every birthday with the knowledge that I am not supposed to be here and with the determination to be here to celebrate the next one.

ACHA participants with life-long significant cardiac disability frequently report taking on professional training and education despite opposition from family or medical professionals, and many achieve high levels of independence and career success.

*Implications for health care providers*

For patients and families who perceive previous surgeries as evidence of a "medical miracle," learning that they have new health problems can be particularly difficult. Conversely, ACHD patients raised with the expectation that they would not live long may have an inappropriately negative view of their expected life span: many are surprised and encouraged to learn that the reported median age of survival in patients who have Eisenmenger's syndrome is into the sixth decade [8]. Those who have repeatedly heard negative health predictions that did not come true may be justifiably skeptical of new information provided by medical professionals. As a result, health care providers should avoid assuming that patients who appear reluctant to accept health information are in denial or unable to comprehend health risks. Care must be taken to establish a supportive and collaborative patient–physician relationship in which patient experiences and medical advice are valued.

**Issue 3: facing the facts and the unknown: patient/physician communication and education**

> [Patient 1] The reason that I thought that I was "fixed" came more from what was not said and because of the old phrase "no news is good news".... It was well known at the time of surgery at the age of six that I may need future surgery, but I was never told, even when I became an adult. I was also never told that things may get worse at all. I was treated as if my heart was not perfect, but there was nothing to worry about. What was said at doctor's appointments was that

everything was fine and that I would need to return in a year or two.

[Patient 2] I wish someone had sat down with me and said, "This is what your heart defect is. These are the consequences and what we are watching for. This is what we know and this is what we don't know. This is what we are doing to help and this is what you can do to optimize your life."

The provision of overly optimistic or overly pessimistic outlooks results in suboptimal knowledge among ACHD patients. ACHA participant reports confirm the existing educational research suggesting that very few adults who have CHD have the knowledge and understanding necessary to ensure appropriate health surveillance behavior and to optimize their health. In their 2001 overview of existing research in patient education, Moons and colleagues [9] reported that between 54% and 76% of patients are able to name their cardiac defect and many ACHA members recall being "drilled" on the name of their diagnosis and previous surgeries by their pediatric care providers, particularly as they reached their teens. Very few, however, can draw or describe their anatomy, and even fewer can identify their specific cardiac issues and the reasons they should return for follow-up care. One study reported that 84% of patients cannot identify the symptoms of heart failure and 92% cannot identify symptoms of endocarditis. Although many patients understand they are expected to return for follow-up care, Moons and colleagues [9] noted that less than half identify the potential for deterioration as a reason for their follow-up visits.

Many factors contribute to the lack of complete knowledge among ACHD patients. Although formal data are lacking, ACHA encounters with cardiology professionals suggest that some health care providers have attitudinal barriers to fully educating CHD survivors about their risks and the need for life-long health surveillance. An often-identified competing goal, particularly in pediatric cardiology, is preventing the potentially detrimental impact of overprotection and limited expectations. Many adults who have complex CHD report strong positive attachment to their pediatric care team based in part on the positive messages they were given: that they were "fine" and they should go out and live a normal life. Many of these same patients, however, took this message so literally that they

left cardiac care—in some cases for decades at a time. Not all survived to return to care.

In working with pediatric and adult cardiologists, ACHA's suggestions to refrain from using words like "fixed" have been met with the assertion that the need to avoid undue anxiety outweighs the need to prepare patients for possible problems that may lie well in the future, and physicians state that information should be given on an as-needed basis. These responses, particularly in the adult context, raise serious ethical concerns. According to the Code of Medical Ethics of the American Medical Association [10]:

It is a fundamental ethical requirement that a physician should at all times deal honestly and openly with patients. Patients have a right to know their past and present medical status and to be free of any mistaken beliefs concerning their conditions.

Although the preferences of ACHD patients have not been studied, patient preference for full disclosure of information regarding other health conditions such as an Alzheimer's disease diagnosis is well documented [11]. It is an accepted concept in bioethics that except in cases in which the patient indicates that she or he does not want to know, respecting the dignity of the patient demands fully sharing health information.

An additional factor directly inhibiting the conveyance of accurate health information is the absence of data on long-term outcomes. Few issues engender as much passion in the ACHD community as the need for more large-scale studies examining long-term outcomes in CHD. ACHD patients report on-going frustration at the number of health questions to which the best answer is "we don't know," particularly when ACHA interactions make clear that the population of complex CHD survivors available for study is large and growing. It is essential that current ACHD patients be identified and studied so that patients and families can benefit from evidence-based practice rather than hopes and suppositions.

Parental responsibility for health care decision making can also influence patient education. During childhood and adolescence, parents are usually considered the "holders of the information," and few patients recall a specific transition of primary medical responsibility from parent to patient. In some families, this transition may not have occurred, and parental fear of risk and loss of control, issues of guilt related to the etiology of the defect, or the patient's own desire to continue within the "safety net" of parental responsibility can result in a continued lack of independence. Frequently, individuals grow up with a "child's understanding" of their cardiac condition (eg, "backwards heart," "hole in the heart"), which may or may not be supplemented with more adult terminology. Some ACHD patients report that their parents' knowledge was also minimal, which may reflect the lack of CHD information at the time or an earlier era of more paternalistic doctor–patient relationships. When ACHD patients ask their parents why they did not tell them more about their defect, typical responses include, "I didn't know," "I did not want to burden you," or "well, since you were fixed, I didn't think the details were important."

Finally, patient behaviors can also contribute to a lack of knowledge. Visits to health care providers can be fraught with worry, and such anxiety interferes with concentration and memory. Concerns that the worst fears will be realized can interfere with the ability to focus on the conversation at hand or to ask for information.

In the absence of accurate information regarding risks and symptoms specific to CHD, many adults who have CHD focus on more widely available information about coronary artery disease symptoms. Many ACHD patients report relying on the absence or presence of chest pain or pressure as their primary indicator of heart health; some believe they are at very high risk of heart attack. Concurrently, symptoms such as fluid retention, racing or pounding heart, and shortness of breath may be ignored or ascribed to aging, weight gain, and anxiety. Discussing children and young adults, Veldtman and colleagues [12] stated, "Illness understanding is poor...and many have an entirely wrong concept of their disease." This lack of understanding also appears prominently in the older ACHD community.

*Implications for health care providers*

Appropriately educating complex CHD survivors requires honesty and humility on the part of the health care providers. The myth of the "fix" and the emphasis on being "normal" must be replaced with an acknowledgment of a life-long health condition and the goal of empowering patients to successfully negotiate life with complex CHD. Although optimism and encouragement are essential, specific assurances such as statements that future surgery is unlikely should be offered only when there are strong supporting data, and those who have undergone recently developed procedures should understand that long-term outcomes, by definition, are as yet unknown. Conversely, negative predictions regarding long-term outcomes should also be made with an acknowledgment that future medical progress is unknown. Past experience in the treatment of CHD suggests that on-going progress will continue to be made in response to today's known problems.

Appropriate ACHD patient education also demands extensive, on-going time and resources, a scarce commodity at many clinics in which existing resources are already stretched thin by the complex medical needs of these highly challenging patients. Having an adequate number of midlevel providers specifically trained in patient education, such as nurses, nurse practitioners, or physician assistants, should be considered a priority. Although high-level technology and medical expertise is essential, equally essential to patient well-being is the availability of relevant information to ensure that they have the knowledge and skills needed to optimize their health and to access care appropriately.

ACHA has defined a "tool kit" of information with which all ACHD patients should be equipped (Box 2). All CHD survivors are required to undertake life-long health surveillance behavior and should be able to identify and describe their defects and previous interventions, observe endocarditis prophylaxis guidelines if appropriate, and obtain cardiac care and testing at recommended intervals. Other specific topics for education might include how to identify and respond to heart failure, arrhythmias, or endocarditis and the known likelihood of future interventions (eg, restenting or valve replacement). It is essential that complex congenital heart defect survivors be instructed on the importance of seeking specialized ACHD care and be given specific strategies and criteria for finding such care. Unless these instructions are made explicit, ACHA experience shows that many complex ACHD patients will seek care from nonpediatric community-level cardiologists or choose cardiologists based on media "health report cards," cardiac center advertising, or name recognition. Patients should also be provided with copies of essential health records such as catheterization and surgical reports and understand that because hospital systems are

Box 2. Adult Congenital Heart Association educational "tool kit"

- Ability to name and describe defect and interventions
- Ability to recognize cardiac symptoms
- Understanding of need for on-going care
- Information on how to find appropriate care
- Understanding of risks particular to defect(s)
- Understanding of risk of CHD recurrence
- Knowledge of appropriate birth control options
- Understanding of pregnancy risks/special needs
- Understanding of appropriate exercise activities
- Access to medical records
- Access to appropriate vocational education
- Access to support and on-going information

legally obligated to keep information for only a limited number of years, it is in their best interest to keep copies of their own health records.

Congenital heart defects are complex and difficult to understand, and a single educational discussion is rarely adequate; patient education must be revisited as many times as needed until a stable understanding is achieved. Patient fears and anxieties should be directly solicited and addressed. There must also be patience and acknowledgment that individuals bring their own limitations for mastering the information. Families in which a parent is still managing health care may require assistance from the health care team to allow the adult patients to take control of their own health care needs. Mastery may also be limited by other barriers such as learning disabilities, impaired cognitive function, and mental illness.

When patients are fully educated about their CHD, not only are they more likely to engage in appropriate health surveillance behavior but they can also use the information to guide life decisions such as when and whether to have children and what career to pursue. When the potential for future problems is significant, patients may wish

to engage as early as possible in activities best undertaken with optimal heart health, such as third-world travel or applying for life insurance. As stated by Feudtner [13], the benefits of appropriate patient education include improved quality of life by increased knowledge and skills, improved self-care, increased adherence to and effectiveness of therapy, better monitoring for possible complications, reduced physical morbidity and risk of mortality, reduced psychosocial stress and anxiety, and enhanced self-esteem, decision-making capacity, and satisfaction with care.

### Issue 4: negotiating the medical system

> [Patient 1] I told them my left and right ventricles were reversed. The cardiologist stated that this did not matter since "the left and right ventricles are the same."
>
> [Patient 2] This is a recurrent conversation that I have with medical staff, especially in the emergency room:
> "Why are you here today"
> "I have a congenital heart defect."
> "Okay, what is it?"
> "A vascular ring."
> "Oh...okay (pause)...so is it metal? When did you have it put in?"
> [Patient 3], "How long have you had a congenital heart defect, Mrs. J"?

When adults who have complex CHD meet and exchange stories, one recurring theme is the misunderstanding and ignorance frequently encountered in the "regular" medical system, especially in the emergency room. Although patients often recount these stories with humor, the realization that one's medical care is in the hands of those who do not understand one's medical condition is terrifying. For many who have complex CHD, establishing safe and effective relationships with their noncardiac care providers involves on-going education and conversations with the ACHD specialists and the patient. For example, adult patients commonly report the need to be vigilant in rejecting inappropriate medications offered by primary care providers. In the context of a medical emergency in the emergency room, patients are faced with medical staff likely to know little or nothing about CHD, and insisting on special care can result in an adversarial situation. For example, one cyanotic patient reported that her increasingly agitated requests for an air filter on her IV line did not result in a filter but did result in the medical staff calling for assistance from the hospital's mental health team.

*Implications for the health care provider*

Patient reports support the importance of the 32nd Bethesda Conference recommendation that all CHD patients be equipped to advocate for their medical needs in urgent situations [14]. Given the rarity and complexity of many CHD diagnoses, ACHD patients should understand that outside of the pediatric and specialized ACHD settings, health care providers are likely to have little or no knowledge of their anatomy and special needs. Although adult patients may wish for a health care system in which they could trust medical professionals to recognize and understand their diagnoses, this is not currently a realistic expectation.

Many patients who have CHD have specific medical "red flags" unique to their defect. Two common examples are the need for filters on intravenous lines for those who have right to left shunting across a defect, and the need for endocarditis testing before antibiotics are given when there is fever of unknown origin. Patients ideally should not only understand these needs but also have the ability to explain them with confidence to medical providers. Patients must serve as their own advocates, at times cajoling health care providers to take appropriate action. Ideally, patients should have a cell phone number or pager number to ensure 24-hour contact with a member of their ACHD team. Even when health records are available, they may not be consulted or the diagnoses and interventions referenced may not be recognized or understood. Reports of resistance or reluctance by the emergency room staff to contacting the ACHD program directly are common. Handing a surprised emergency room physician a cell phone connected to an ACHD specialist can be quite effective.

In addition to primary care and emergency room providers, ACHD clinic staff should be prepared to educate the teams of providers during hospitalizations. At times, escorting the patient from site to site through hospitalizations is necessary to ensure no errors occur at any step of the way. In the words of Dr. Jane Somerville [15],

> These are a precious group of patients.... Half the avoidable deaths occurred in those who were well, leading normal lives without symptoms or with mild disability...errors of management are being made at all levels in the care of the GUCH [ACHD] patient.

## Issue 5: invisible disabilities

> [Patient 1] What's frustrating is that because you don't have some visible handicap like the loss of limbs, people seem to think you're faking, or they forget you have it, or something. And who of us wants to keep reminding people they have heart problems? I hate saying it, period.

> [Patient 2] When I have a bad day, my husband accuses me of making it up.

Like other invisible disabilities, cardiac health problems such as heart failure and arrhythmias can produce a particular set of issues with family and the larger community. ACHD patients commonly report family or friends who imply that their problems are "in their head" or insist that changes to work, childcare, or household responsibilities are not necessary. Reports of difficulties at work related to misunderstandings about a patient's physical limitations are also common. Because ACHD patients may appear to be well, requests for time off or other accommodations, such as adjustments in work schedule or responsibilities, may be met with skepticism or accusations of dishonesty. Many ACHD patients using handicapped parking stickers report being challenged by bystanders who believe they are parking illegitimately. Responses to this particular situation can be creative: one patient developed a false limp to use in the parking lot, another started lifting her shirt and showing her scars to all challengers.

*Implications for health care providers*

Health care providers are encouraged to explicitly ask patients about their support systems and the level of understanding these people have about the patients' limitations and to address the stresses these issues can cause. Patients report that direct communication between spouse or family members and care providers can be extremely helpful, particularly when family members are encouraged to ask questions and raise independent concerns. Questions about workplace difficulties should also be included; when appropriate, supports such as workplace letters and documentation of health status can be offered.

## Issue 6: confronting mortality

> [Patient 1] I found out how serious things were when I changed doctors at the age of twenty-five and found out I needed heart surgery again...I was

scared, angry, and felt completely alone. Since my mother knew all along that I may need more surgery and did not tell me, I did not trust her to tell me the truth.... At the time I was seeing new doctors and didn't know exactly what to ask them.

[Patient 2] I was furious—I kept saying, "but they told me I would be fine!" and they kept saying, "You knew you had this condition. You're actually lucky to have lived this long."

For many ACHD patients, new health information comes not in the context of a planned transition or educational process but at the onset of new health problems. Despite the fact that most patients have always known that they have CHD, the onset of new problems can be analogous to the onset of any adult-onset, new, potentially fatal condition. Those who discover that information on future health risks was withheld may have an additional layer of anger and a sense of having been deceived or betrayed. Particularly difficult situations include facing difficult treatment decisions, referral for surgery, or being told that "nothing more can be done" [16]. Psychosocial research has found that the manner in which adults who have CHD cope with their disease is impacted by environmental factors (eg, friends and family), experiences with medical treatment and health care providers, and personal attributes (eg, whether they believe outcomes reflect personal actions or external factors) [17]. For participants in ACHA, a primary coping strategy is often getting peer support from those who have faced similar challenges, and many report these interactions to be profoundly helpful.

Although CHD is best considered a chronic condition, new problems can dramatically change the patient's experience and outlook. It is unfortunate that the gap between patient and care provider may become particularly acute at this time. Health care providers may indicate annoyance with the patient's distress and lack of understanding or imply that the patient "should have known" that future health problems were likely.

*Implications for health care providers*

The congenital heart patient experiencing new, serious health problems should be offered the same compassion, education, and support resources that would be offered adults newly diagnosed with other life-threatening conditions. Medical professionals working with adults who have CHD are encouraged to be particularly respectful and sensitive during these times. Although health care providers may be surprised by a patient's lack of previous knowledge, it is never appropriate to imply that the patient has been in denial. At no time should patients facing life-threatening health problems be told by their health care team that they are lucky or they should be grateful. It is appropriate to refer patients who have significant difficulties managing these situations to mental health professionals who are able to provide emotional support in addition to specific coping strategies. Opportunities for peer support should also be offered.

### Issue 7: what is "normal"?

[Patient 1] I grew up knowing I had brown eyes, brown hair, and a backwards heart.

[Patient 2] I hate when they ask, "How do you feel compared with a normal person?" I always want to say, "How the hell would I know?"

ACHD survivors report widely variable childhood experiences that were influenced by many factors including health status, family styles and structure, and personalities. Multiple psychosocial studies, however, have suggested that feeling "different" is a common experience among patients who have CHD [16–20]. This feeling is not surprising because the experiences of most of these individuals are different from those of children born without congenital heart defects. Examples of the experiences that many "heart kids" share include cardiology visits, cardiac testing, taking medications, school activity restrictions, hospitalizations, interventions, and having a scar. Depending on health status, reported challenges may also include frequent school absences, academic struggles due to absence or illness, or the inability to participate in childhood activities such as riding a bike or playing tag. For the small minority of patients who experience on-going significant cyanosis, reports of teasing and negative attention brought on by having blue lips and clubbed fingers are common; research by Horner and colleagues [16] reported that most boys who have cyanotic CHD describe teasing, rejection, and distressing nicknames.

Research suggests that approximately one fourth of adults who have CHD recall parental overprotection during childhood and adolescence [19,21,22], and the theme of parental overprotection is echoed in the recollections of some ACHA members. It must be emphasized, however, that this behavior does not reflect that of all or even most parents. Congenital heart survivors report a wide range of parenting styles, including parents who were risk-taking, casual, or neglectful.

[Patient 3] Even when I was the "bluest kid in class," I played baseball, basketball, football, and most other kids' games. My mother was determined that if I had a short time to live, she would allow me to live it doing the things I enjoyed doing.

[Patient 4] I was raised by narcissistic parents who had little regard for anyone other than themselves and what they felt like doing in the moment. [I had] heart and lung problems in a house full of heavy smokers and drinkers.

Such neglect can have devastating consequences; for example, some patients who have Eisenmenger's syndrome struggle with the knowledge that their parents' failure to obtain prompt medical care was a central factor in their compromised health and limited options. ACHA participant experiences also suggest that given the right education and support, even the most overprotected "heart kid" can become an independent and effective self-advocate.

Although many interviewees in qualitative research studies describe striving for normality [17,18], many of the ACHD patients encountered by the ACHA express irritation with the word *normal*, particularly in the context of their health and experience. One of the first questions parents of children who have heart defects typically ask ACHD patients is, "Are you able to have a normal life?" For those diagnosed as children, however, having a heart defect is normal. For some patients, their CHD has or will involve many limitations and challenges; for others, very few. If normal is defined as typical, then being normal is not an appropriate goal for those who have complex CHD. Part of the maturational process identified by many adults who have CHD is coming to terms with the challenges presented by their heart defect and realizing that the concept of normal is an artifice and having limitations is the human condition.

[Patient 5] We all are "dealt a hand" in life—heart defect, dyslexia, quick temper, tone deaf, drug-addicted mother, shy, bossy, born poor, diabetic, etcetera. Some of us just know sooner than others what our cards are.

[Patient 6] I can't...get caught up in the idea that life has been "unfair" to me. Especially as there are so many other ways life could have been so much more unfair.... Do I wonder what it would be like

to spring out of bed and go jogging? Sure! But we all wonder about the things others have that we don't.

Although adults in the CHD cohort showed significant physical dysfunction on objective testing, Moons [23] found that adults who have CHD assess their health status to be equal to that of their heart-healthy peers. For some, this may be because their "normal function" has always been subnormal; for others, it may be that the dysfunction they are now experiencing developed over time, with the patient unknowingly adjusting his or her behavior to the new level of function. Overall, it suggests that most adults who have CHD are content with their abilities and do not experience diminished physical capabilities as a loss.

Examining the language that CHD survivors use to describe their condition also illuminates the way that many see CHD as part of their self-identity. Many adults who have CHD strongly object to the use of the word *disease* to describe their anatomy because it implies that they were "born diseased." For the layperson, disease often connotes contagion, and "heart disease" is often used as a synonym for coronary artery disease. One of the most common complaints of heart defect survivors is being confused with elderly heart attack victims. For some, the term *defect* is also seen as offensive because it implies that they themselves are "defective." It would be the rare patient who has cancer or acquired heart disease who would take criticism of their disease personally, but this generalization from defective heart to defective self illustrates that many of those who grew up with CHD see their heart as an essential component of themselves.

The most common term used by patients to describe their heart is the more neutral phrase *heart condition*, thereby referring to the heart's static, anatomic reality. When patients encounter health problems, a distinction is often made between the heart defect itself and the consequences of the defect (ie, heart failure, pulmonary hypertension, arrhythmia, and endocarditis).

Patients who have experienced life-long significant cardiac disability may struggle with surgical decisions that offer the potential of significant functional improvement, often making comments such as, "but I do fine" or "but I'm not that blue." Patients who experience significant functional improvement (eg, after Fontan revision) often comment that they had no idea that they could feel this well.

*Implications for health care providers*

One challenge for health care providers and educators is to use language that does not alienate the patients but accurately reflects the reality of their conditions and on-going health care needs. A component of some patients' rejection of the term *congenital heart disease* may be lack of understanding or denial of the serious health risks and the often progressive dysfunction that can come with CHD. The usefulness of the term *congenital heart disease* is limited by its generality; each defect has its own unique anatomy and concerns, and most health problems involved in CHD can be best discussed in the context of a specific defect. Explaining things in defect-specific language (ie, "people born with tetralogy of Fallot") reinforces a patient's knowledge of his or her own diagnosis and helps support the key concept that all congenital heart defects are different. In printed patient materials, ACHA uses the term *congenital heart defect*, which avoids the negative overtones potentially associated with the word *disease* and the vagueness and potential euphemism of the word *condition*.

Given the well-documented inability of ACHD patients to accurately assess their own physical function, objective measurements of functional capacity such as exercise testing with maximum $Vo_2$ determination is essential. Discussions of function should focus on relative changes or stability for the individual and should inform decisions about the need for therapeutic changes. Results discussed and compared with normal function may be useful for some as general markers but may raise significant issues for the individual and do not necessarily inform the discussion in a frame of reference that enables the individual to consider his or her stability or decline in functional capacity. The importance of reaching maximum potential rather than attaining "normality" must be emphasized. When discussing potential interventions such as surgery, there must be an open exchange between the provider and the individual regarding reasonable expectations for results and improvement in functional capacity. Conversations with others who have undergone similar surgeries can help patients understand potential functional outcomes.

**Issue 8: the gift of congenital heart disease**

[Patient 1] I like who I am and the people I've met along the way. I am far less shallow and way more empathetic than I would have been without CHD. Last month when I went snowshoeing in the mountains, the sky was bluer, the mountains grander, and the company finer because I spent last summer chained to the flatlands with arrhythmia. I live in gratitude more because I know some days are not so good. Life is far more precious knowing the alternatives that I've faced at times.

[Patient 2] I know every day when I look in the mirror and see my scars that I am a living miracle and have been blessed by God more times than I can count.

[Patient 3] My father...told me at an early age that..."you are different. The demands on you throughout childhood and adulthood will be different than everyone else's. Therefore, this is what we're going to do..." He taught me that I couldn't do blue collar work. And because of that, I needed to be better than the next person at whatever I did. He taught me to invest in the stock market at age seven. He taught me accounting at age nine. I attended my first shareholder's meeting at age ten. He taught me to exploit my assets and not dwell on my limitations. He gave me an extra skill set that he did not give my brother or sister because he felt the demands on me would be higher.

Although we have focused on the concerns and frustrations faced by many adults with CHD, it is also important to highlight the fact that many long-term survivors report benefits from their experiences with CHD. Adults who have CHD often report positive and negative childhood associations: for example, yearly cardiology visits might bring not only time alone with parents but also rare treats such as train rides, hotel visits, new toys, and meals out. For those uninterested in athletics, being excused from running laps can be a privilege and make one the envy of one's fellow nonathletes. Many adult patients report jealousy from brothers and sisters because they received "special" treatment growing up. The experience of facing fear and overcoming medical adversity can yield life-long resilience and the ability to pursue long-term goals. It is common for ACHD patients to report that they were the first in their family to go to college, some using vocational services funding offered because of their cardiac disability.

In recent years, disability researchers have identified a large gap between how those who are nondisabled perceive the quality of life of those who have disabling conditions (which is uniformly negative) and how those who have such conditions perceive themselves. Moons' [23] finding of positive health assessment in the CHD community is echoed in numerous studies that find that patient perception of personal health status and abilities in a wide variety of disabling conditions is at odds with objective health status. Multiple studies have found that most of those living with significant disabilities report that their quality of life is good or excellent [24,25]. One study examining this phenomenon identified the following factors as key to perceived high quality of life with disability: acknowledgment of one's impairment, preserved control over mind and body, the ability to perform expected roles, a "can-do" attitude, finding a purpose and meaning in life, having a spiritual foundation, social connections, and feeling satisfied with one's capabilities in the context of one's particular health condition [26]. These same key factors are often referenced by CHD survivors.

Other "benefit finding" studies report similar findings. For example, in a qualitative study of 16 stroke survivors, 63% identified positive consequences in the domains of increased social relationships, increased health awareness, change in religious life, personal growth, and altruism [27]. Moons and colleagues [28] reported that ACHD patients indicated they placed less emphasis on financial means and material well-being than their heart-healthy peers. Many ACHD survivors echo the opinions expressed in *What's Your Expiry Date?*, the recent book by Canadian ACHD advocate Patrick Mathieu [29], which describes how the on-going awareness of one's mortality can lead to clarity of purpose, better decision-making, and a deep appreciation for life.

*Implications for health care providers*

Because most health care providers see their patients only within a medical setting, opportunities to observe the gifts of CHD and the resilience of CHD survivors may be limited. ACHD patients often comment that because of the anxiety and stress raised in the medical setting, their health care providers tend to see them at "their worst." The appropriate goal of medicine is to identify health problems, cure disease, and relieve symptoms; therefore, there are few opportunities to discuss contentment in the face of limitations. As noted by Moons and colleagues [30], however, an essential component of assessing long-term CHD outcomes is creating quality-of-life indicators that accurately assess the patient's own contentment and experience rather than his or her ability to function normally. Health care providers working with the pediatric community are

encouraged to remind parents that health status and functional capacity are different from quality of life. Health care providers can help avoid inappropriately negative projections by helping parents understand that significant health challenges in no way preclude a high quality of life and can build resilience, optimism, and contentment.

For patients reporting a poor quality of life, potential interventions that address the factors listed earlier might include increasing patient understanding of their disease to improve a sense of mastery, helping to identify core functional goals and strategies to achieve these goals, or providing opportunities to meet others facing similar health challenges. When appropriate, referral to mental health professionals for assessment and treatment of potential depression and for therapeutic intervention should be made. It should not be assumed that poor quality of life is a necessary corollary of significant cardiac disability.

**Issue 9: the importance of patient associations**

In the last 15 years, numerous associations for adult survivors of CHD have been formed throughout Europe, Australia, Canada, and the United States: an interactive world map listing international ACHD groups is available at www.worldcongenitalheart.org. The psychosocial benefits of patients interacting with others who share their health challenges should not be underestimated; opportunities for peer support help address many of the issues identified in this article.

In addition to offering peer support, ACHD patient associations can play a seminal role in addressing the many existing challenges facing long-term survivors of CHD. Patient organizations in other diseases, such as the National Marfan Foundation, the Cystic Fibrosis Foundation, and the Pulmonary Hypertension Association, demonstrate the efficacy of such groups in promoting research, establishing care guidelines, and providing resources to their communities. When patients speak directly about their own experiences and advocate for their own life-long needs, they have unique power and impact. Participation in advocacy can be a transformative experience for the patients and family members involved: for example, many patient and family participants in ACHA's 2005 National ACHD Lobby Day commented that in educating lawmakers about the unique needs of the ACHD community, life-long frustrations were translated into effective action.

Table 1
Adult congenital heart disease patient association challenges and contributions

| Challenges facing ACHD patients | ACHA program |
| --- | --- |
| Social isolation and lack of support | Online discussion board<br>Opportunities to meet other ACHD patients |
| Public awareness and finding "the lost" | Media campaigns<br>National ACHD Lobby Day |
| Lack of patient education | Patient/family conferences<br>Patient/family Newsletter<br>Online information |
| Access to medical records<br>Access to appropriate care | Print and Electronic Personal Health Passport<br>ACHD Clinic Directory<br>Dissemination of existing ACHD care guidelines<br>ACHA-sponsored Continuing Medical Education programs |
| Lack of ACHD research | Promotion of national ACHD registry<br>Sponsorship of national ACHD research symposium |

As an example of what patient associations can undertake, Table 1 lists the key challenges identified by ACHA and the initiatives addressing these challenges. A number of these are collaborative efforts: for example, the National ACHD Clinic Directory is a joint project between ACHA and ISACCD, and ACHA's 2005 National ACHD Lobby Day involved numerous partners including the American College of Cardiology, the Congenital Heart Information Network, and the Children's Heart Foundation. Such collaboration is directly addressed in the 32nd Bethesda Conference Report, which calls for the establishment of a national patient advocacy organization and collaborations between patients, families, health care providers, federal agencies, and professional organizations to promote the provision of long-term care to the CHD community.

A major triumph of twentieth century medicine was the success of childhood interventions for CHD and the creation of the first large cohort of ACHD survivors. A major challenge for the twenty-first century is how to address the long-term surveillance and health care needs created by the transformation of complex CHD from a fatal to a life-long condition. As the primary life-long stakeholders, the patients themselves must continue to be central to this effort, and their perspective must continue to inform the development of a cardiac care system that meets the needs of the CHD community.

Just as ACHD patients as a group must remain central in the design and provision of care systems for CHD survivors, each individual ACHD patient must be equipped to play a central role in his or her own life-long cardiac care. Due to the novelty and rarity of these conditions among adults, ACHD patients are called on to self-advocate with medical professionals who have little knowledge of their disease and to negotiate adult roles in a community that has little awareness of congenital heart defects. As described earlier, many ACHA participants report barriers to care and well-being that might have been avoided or ameliorated with better and more honest communication, more accurate information, or more insight and assistance from previous health care providers. For each issue identified in this article, the authors have outlined implications for the ACHD health professional and made recommendations for best practices. Table 1 summarizes specific behaviors to avoid and best practices to promote. Overall, the authors' goal is to help ensure that every ACHD survivor has the tools she or he needs to maximize his or her life span, functional status, and quality of life.

## Appendix 1

### Classification of congenital heart defects

*Group 1: congenital heart disease of mild complexity*

Native conditions:

Isolated congenital aortic valve disease
Isolated congenital mitral valve disease
(except parachute valve, cleft leaflet)

Isolated PFO/small atrial septal defect
Isolated small ventricular septal defect
Mild pulmonic stenosis

Repaired conditions:

Previously ligated or occluded patent ductus arteriosus
Repaired secundum or sinus venosus atrial septal defect without residua
Repaired ventricular septal defect without residua

*Group 2: congenital heart disease of moderate complexity*

Aorto-left ventricular fistulae
Anomalous pulmonary venous drainage
Atrioventricular canal/septal defects
Ostium primum atrial septal defect
Coarctation of the aorta
Ebstein's anomaly
Infundibular right ventricular outflow obstruction
Patent ductus arteriosus (not closed)
Pulmonary valve regurgitation (moderate to severe)
Pulmonary valve stenosis (moderate to severe)
Sinus of Valsalva fistula/aneurysm
Sinus venosus atrial septal defects
Subvalvular or supravalvar aortic stenosis
Tetralogy of Fallot
Ventricular septal defect with
    Absent valve or valves
    Coarctation of the aorta
    Mitral disease
    Right ventricular outflow tract obstruction
    Straddling tricuspid/mitral valve
    Subaortic stenosis

*Group 3: congenital heart disease of great complexity*

Conduits, valved, or nonvalved
Cyanotic CHD (all forms)
Double-outlet ventricle
Eisenmenger's syndrome
Fontan procedure
Mitral atresia
Functionally single ventricle
Pulmonary atresia (all forms)
Pulmonary vascular obstructive disease
Transposition of the great arteries
Congenitally corrected transposition of the great arteries

Tricuspid atresia
Truncus arteriosus/hemitruncus
Other abnormalities of atrioventricular or ventriculoarterial connection not included above (ie, crisscross heart, isomerism, heterotaxy syndromes)

## References

[1] Webb GD, Williams R. 32nd Bethesda Conference: "care of the adult with congenital heart disease. J Am Coll Cardiol 2001;37(5):1161–98.
[2] Warnes CA. The adult with congenital heart disease: born to be bad? J Am Coll Cardiol 2005;46(1):1–8.
[3] Deanfield J, Thaulow E, Warnes CA, et al. Management of grown up congenital heart disease: the Task Force on the Management of Grown Up Congenital Heart Disease of the European Society of Cardiology. Eur Heart J 2003;24(11):1035–84.
[4] Connelly MS, Webb GD, Somerville J, et al. Canadian consensus conference on adult congenital heart disease 1996. Can J Cardiol 1998;14(3):395–452.
[5] Wernovsky G, Rome JJ, Tabbutt S, et al. Guidelines for outpatient management of complex congenital heart disease. Congenit Heart Dis 2006;1(1–2):10–26.
[6] Kidd L, Driscoll D, Gersony W. Second natural history study of congenital heart defects: results of treatment of patients with ventricular septal defects. Circulation 1993;87(2 Suppl):138–51.
[7] Reid GJ, Irvine MJ, McCrindle BW, et al. Prevalence and correlates of successful transfer from pediatric to adult health care among a cohort of young adults with complex congenital heart defects. Pediatrics 2004;113(3 Pt 1):e197–205.
[8] Cantor WJ, Harrison DA, Moussadji JS, et al. Determinants of survival and length of survival in adults with Eisenmenger syndrome. Am J Cardiol 1999;84(6):677–81.
[9] Moons P, De Volder E, Budts W, et al. What do adult patients with congenital heart disease know about their disease, treatment, and prevention of complications? A call for structured patient education. Heart 2001;86(1):74–80.
[10] American Medical Association. E-8.12. Patient information page. Available at: http://www.ama-assn.org/ama/pub/category/8497.html. Accessed May 9, 2006.
[11] Erde EL, Nadal EC, Scholl TO. On truth-telling and the diagnosis of Alzheimer's disease. J Fam Pract 1988;24(4):401–6.
[12] Veldtman GR, Matley SL, Kendall L, et al. Illness understanding in children and adolescents with heart disease. West J Med 2001;174(3):173–4.

[13] Feudtner C. What are the goals of patient education? Heart 2000;84:395–7.

[14] Landzberg MJ, Murphy DJ Jr, Davidson WR, et al. Task force 4: organization of delivery systems for adults with congenital heart disease. J Am Coll Cardiol 2001;37(5):1161–98.

[15] Somerville J. Near misses and disasters in the treatment of grown-up congenital heart patients. J R Soc Med 1997;90:124–7.

[16] Horner T, Lieberthson R, Jellinek MS. Psychosocial profile of adults with complex congenital heart disease. Mayo Clin Proc 2000;75(1):31–6.

[17] Tong EM, Sparacino PS, Messias DK, et al. Growing up with congenital heart disease: the dilemmas of adolescents and young adults. Cardiol Young 1998; 8(3):303–9.

[18] Claessens P, Moons P, de Casterle BD, et al. What does it mean to live with a congenital heart disease? A qualitative study on the lived experiences of adult patients. Eur J Cardiovasc Nurs 2005;4(1):3–10.

[19] McMurray R, Kendall L, Parson JM, et al. A life less ordinary: growing up and coping with congenital heart disease. Coron Health Care 2001;5(1):51–7.

[20] Gantt LT. Growing up heartsick: the experiences of young women with congenital heart disease. Health Care Women Int 1992;13(3):241–8.

[21] Brandhagen DJ, Feldt RH, Williams DE. Long-term psychologic implications of congenital heart disease: a 25-year follow-up. Mayo Clin Proc 1991; 66(5):474–9.

[22] Arnett JJ. Emerging adulthood: a theory of development form the late teens through the twenties. Am Psychol 2000;55(5):469–80.

[23] Moons P, Van Deyk K, De Bleser L, et al. Links quality of life and health status in adults with congenital heart disease: a direct comparison with healthy counterparts. Eur J Cardiovasc Prev Rehabil 2006;13(3):407–13.

[24] Albrecht GL, Higgins P. Rehabilitation success: the interrelationships of multiple criteria. J Health Soc Behav 1997;18:36–45.

[25] Weinberg N. Another perspective: attitudes of people with disabilities. In: Attitudes toward persons with disabilities. New York: Springer; 1998. p. 141–53.

[26] Albrecht GL, Devlieger PJ. The disability paradox: high quality of life against all odds. Soc Sci Med 1999;48:977–88.

[27] Gillen G. Positive consequences of surviving a stroke. Am J Occup Ther 2005;59(3):346–50.

[28] Moons P, Van Deyk K, De Geest S, et al. Is the severity of congenital heart disease associated with the quality of life and perceived health of adult patients? Heart 2005;91(9):1193–8.

[29] Mathieu P. What's Your Expiry Date? Ontario, Canada: Patrick Mathieu Unlimited; 2005.

[30] Moons P, Van Deyk K, Marquet K. Individual quality of life in adults with congenital heart disease: a paradigm shift. Eur Heart J 2005;26(3): 298–307.

ELSEVIER
SAUNDERS

Cardiol Clin 24 (2006) 531–556

CARDIOLOGY
CLINICS

# The Role of Cardiac Catheterization in Adult Congenital Heart Disease

Peter McLaughlin, MD, FRCP(C)[a,*], Lee Benson, MD, FRCP(C)[b],
Eric Horlick, MD, FRCP(C)[c]

[a]*Peterborough Regional Health Centre, Peterborough, ON, Canada*
[b]*Division of Cardiology, Hospital for Sick Children, Toronto, ON, Canada*
[c]*University Health Network, Toronto, ON, Canada*

The purpose of this article is to define the role of cardiac catheterization in modern adult congenital heart disease (ACHD) facilities. The role of heart catheterization continues to evolve as the sophistication of cardiac MRI and CT improves and the breadth of interventional catheter techniques widens dramatically. This task is approached from four perspectives. The first is the planning of the procedure, including consideration of the information required, the potential pitfalls to be anticipated, and the equipment needed for the procedure. The second perspective is the performance of the procedure, including the essential points related to the sample run, coronary arteriography, chamber angiography, and angiography of selected specific lesions. The third perspective is the current role of heart catheterization with a consideration of the impact of echo, MRI, and CT on indications for catheterization procedures and a brief look at today's interventional procedures. Finally, new and emerging interventions are considered and speculation is given to the future role of diagnostic heart catheterization in patients who have ACHD.

## Planning the procedure

The quality and usefulness of the diagnostic information yielded by a catheterization procedure can be related directly to the quality of the planning and preparation undertaken before the

catheterization study and the knowledge base and experience of the operators. Operators must have a thorough understanding of the anatomy and physiology of congenital cardiac defects, the potential defects associated with the primary defect, the therapeutic options for the defect under investigation, and the information surgeons or interventionalists require if patients are to be referred for treatment. They need to know

What information is absolutely essential to establish a diagnosis or plan treatment;
What information is useful to obtain but is not critical; and
What information is redundant and already available from other imaging studies.

This information, combined with a discussion with adult congenital cardiac clinicians who are leading patient care, provides the questions that must be answered. When such thought and preparation has been done before the procedure, catheterization can be performed in the most efficient manner, minimizing radiation exposure, length of the procedure, and volume of contrast media.

Preprocedural preparation includes a review of the echo Doppler information, CT scanning, cardiac MRI, and functional cardiac testing, such as perfusion imaging, if available. Operators then understand the anatomy, what is known, and what information must be obtained for the assessment of particular patients.

*What information is essential?*

Not uncommonly, studies in some complex cases become unnecessarily long or, perhaps worse,

---

* Corresponding author. 1 Hospital Drive, Peterborough, ON, Canada K9J 7C6.
*E-mail address:* pmclaugh@prhc.on.ca (P. McLaughlin).

are completed without a key piece of information having been obtained. The most common essential information concerns the pulmonary vasculature: the pulmonary artery pressures and resistance, the reactivity of the pulmonary vasculature, and shunt calculations. If access to the pulmonary artery is difficult, this may mean prolongation of the procedure, but time invested here may be far more valuable than recapturing other data already clear from other diagnostic testing. Similarly, the temptation may occur to defer coronary angiography after a difficult procedure in young adults in the precoronary age group, missing the opportunity to detect a relevant congenital anomaly of the coronary circulation.

*What catheters to use and the sequence of events*

Prepared operators go into a cardiac catheter laboratory with a clear idea of which catheters are likely to be most helpful and the sequence they wish to follow to obtain the information. For example, it may be useful to begin the right heart catheterization with a steerable catheter, such as a Goodale-Lubin catheter to sample for oxygen saturation and probe for atrial septal defects (ASDs) and anomalous venous drainage, then change to a balloon-tipped angiocatheter to reach the pulmonary artery through a difficult right ventricular outflow tract. Operators are chagrined if they realize they have reached the pulmonary artery but have forgotten to obtain all the oximetry samples and pressures on the way up. They then face the choice of compromising the saturation run and pressures with some delayed postangiographic measurements or having to withdraw the catheter, obtain the measurements, and re-enter the pulmonary artery, adding to fluoroscopy and procedure time.

To summarize, make a mental checklist at the beginning of the procedure outlining which hemodynamic information must be obtained, which chamber and great vessel angiography must be done, whether or not the coronary anatomy must be determined, which catheters are most useful, and the sequence to be followed throughout the procedure.

**What can go wrong**

The common problems with cardiac catheterization studies of adult patients who have congenital cardiac disease relate to

Prolonged catheterization time and contrast used

Inadequate, missing, or nondiagnostic information obtained
Redundant information obtained
Catheter complications

Many of these problems can be minimized with planning and consultation with clinicians and surgeons involved in patients' care. Most of these procedures can be expected to take substantially more time to complete than the usual right and left heart procedures in patients who have coronary or valvular heart disease, particularly if an unexpected finding arises during the procedure. Keep in mind, however, the key questions as the catheterization progresses.

1. Have the diagnosis and best form of treatment been established?
2. Do I have the essential information required to establish the diagnosis, define the anatomy, define the physiology, define the presence or absence of associated anomalies, and provide the surgeon/interventionalist with the information required?
3. If not, must this information be obtained at this procedure, or can noninvasive testing obtain equivalent or better information?
4. How much contrast has been used so far in this procedure? Has the patient been prehydrated adequately?
5. How is the patient tolerating the procedure—if poorly, should the procedure be terminated with plans for a second procedure to obtain any further essential data?
6. Are there comorbidities that might add to the risk of a complication and, if so, what are the potential preventive measures (eg, erythrocytosis increases the risk of catheter clotting, so more frequent flushing is required)?
7. Am I collecting the information in the right sequence (eg, Have I acquired all the pressure and oximetry samples on the way up to the pulmonary artery? Have I acquired all the hemodynamic measurements before proceeding to angiography?)?

Although no procedure can ever be entirely risk-free, taking these precautions lessens the chance of problems occurring.

**Equipment for interventional cardiac catheterization**

As in adult coronary interventions, a considerable amount of equipment is required to address the varied lesions that present in the catheterization laboratory. Unlike coronary angioplasty and stenting, however, the different types of devices, wires, catheters, embolization, and retrieval equipment can be vast when addressing congenital heart lesions. It is challenging especially in pediatric laboratories, where the inventory has to further address varied patient sizes. If money is not an issue (at the rare institution), then it is possible to keep everything in stock. If finances are limited, then rational stocking of the laboratory is needed, as a laboratory cannot have everything but must have the equipment to cover most of the procedures. There are three principles of inventory management: PLANNING, PLANNING, and PLANNING.

The types of equipment needed to cover most interventional cases include sheaths, guide wires, catheters, guiding catheters, balloons, coils, occlusion devices, stents, covered stents, and retrieval kits.

*Sheaths*

A selection of sheaths from 4- to 12-Fr is required. If the technique of coarctation stenting is offered, a 14-Fr system is needed (for covered stent implantation). Rarely do operators need an 18-Fr sheath. Short percutaneous sheaths to long transseptal lengths should be available. There are various Mullins-type sheaths, and they should be purchased with radio-opaque tip markers (Fig. 1). Additionally, some operators find it helpful to have kink-resistant long sheaths, but this may not be an issue in adult patients, as the intravascular curves are gentler.

*Guide wires*

A selection of guide wires, with sizes from 0.01 in to 0.03 in, in lengths from 50 cm to 260 cm, is needed (Fig. 2). They should be super-floppy,

ordinary, super-stiff, and glide wire (eg, Terumo) varieties. The so-called "Amplatzer stiff" and "ultra-stiff" guide wires (0.025 in to 0.038 in) are found invaluable for stabilizing balloons across high flow lesions and during stent implantation.

*Catheters*

A variety of catheters is required. Basic configurations, such as the multipurpose (Goodale-Lubin), pigtails, NIH, cobra, Judkins coronary, and Multitrack (NuMed, Hopkinton, New York) should be available. Infusion catheters (such as the Tracker-18) should be available. Tapered and nontapered catheters, guiding catheters, and balloon wedge (end-hole) and angiographic (side-hole) catheters, such as the Berman catheters (Critikon), are the foundation of any interventional laboratory (Fig. 3).

A comprehensive stock of catheters is not needed. Operators should choose an appropriate selection and become familiar with their use. The more complex the case mix, the greater the variety of catheters needed.

*Miscellaneous equipment*

Transseptal needles, using the Mullins technique, occasionally are required to enter the left heart or perforate an atretic vascular structure. For adults, a single length of transseptal needle can be stocked, but the needle must fit the long sheath dilator. Additionally, the hub of the dilator should be such that when the needle and hub are engaged, only 2 or 3 cm of the needle are exposed from the tip.

*Balloons*

Although adult interventional cardiologists are experienced with a variety of coronary balloons for primary angioplasty and as a platform for stent delivery, the form and function of the balloons used in interventions that focus on

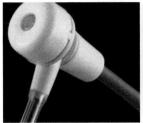 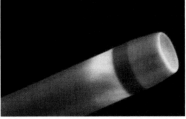

Fig. 1. The left panel is a photo of the side-arm bleed-back tap on a Mullins-type long sheath, whereas the right panel shows the radio-opaque marker tip, which is most useful when initially positioning the sheath and when directing a balloon stent toward the target lesion.

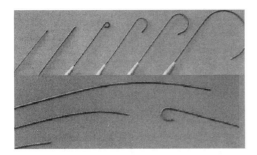

Fig. 2. Wires of various curves.

a congenital heart patient population are different regarding size, length, design, and material. Furthermore, many of the balloons used initially were produced not for intracardiac or pulmonary applications but for peripheral angioplasty.

Low-pressure balloons (eg, Tyshak II, Z-Med [II], NuMed) are available in a range of sizes, many on 4- to 6-Fr shafts. They are advantageous especially because of their rapid deflation rates, which limit the time an outflow tract is occluded during a procedure. High-pressure balloons also come in a range of sizes and lengths from several manufacturers (NuMed-Mullins high pressure balloons, Cordis Johnson & Johnson). Most balloons can be used as platforms for stent delivery. The NuMed BIB (balloon in a balloon) is popular

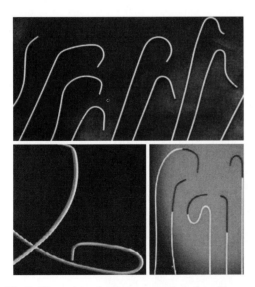

Fig. 3. The variety of catheter curves is endless. The authors find the most useful to be the Judkins right coronary, multipurpose, and cobra shapes. Operators must determine their own preferences for each type of vascular structure that must be traversed.

for controlled expansion and is useful especially for stent delivery. Despite the enormous selection that is available, a large number of different makes of balloons is not needed (Figs. 4 and 5).

*Embolization equipment*

In patients who have congenital heart disorders, standard embolization devices, such as coils, have, in many instances, been supplanted by the application of device implants designed for other locations and indications, such as ductal, atrial, and patent foramen ovale (PFO) defect occluders.

*Coils*

For several years, the Gianturco free release coil (Cook) has been the primary device for peripheral embolization, and it remains the single most used implant in congenital lesions (patent arterial duct, aortopulmonary collaterals, and acquired venovenous collaterals). Controlled release coils (where release is dependent on an active maneuver from the operator), however, offer a safer implant, especially in higher flow lesions or areas where precise coil implantation is critical. A large variety of sizes, lengths, and shapes is available, from various suppliers. Additionally, a selection of guiding and delivery catheters (eg, Tracker-18; Cook) to allow coil embolization of very tortuous vessels should be available (Fig. 6).

Controlled release coils offer an additional advantage for they can be retrieved and repositioned before release. Some coil formats use an electrolytic detachment, whereas others a mechanical release mechanism. Such coils are atraumatic and result in no damage to the vessel. They offer low radial friction within the delivery catheter lumen for easy placement. For an effective occlusion, a dense mass of coils is needed. As such, they take a longer time to form a thrombus than feathered steel coils. The detachable controlled release coils are made of platinum 0.018-in and 0.011-in wire. They are introduced through a Tracker-18 catheter with a simple introducer system. Several coil shapes are available.

*Atrial and ventricular septal devices*

There are several devices clinically available for closure of secundum atrial and ventricular septal defects (primary muscular) (Fig. 7). The Amplatzer (AGA Medical, Golden Valley, Minnesota), CardioSEAL or Starflex (NMT Medical), and Helex (Gore Medical) are a few of the devices approved for clinical use. What is kept in inventory

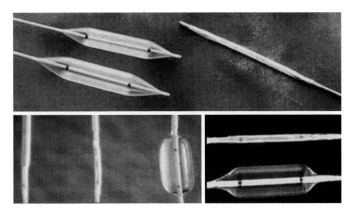

Fig. 4. Various balloons used for stent delivery and vessel/valve angioplasty.

depends on operator experience, and the range and number of defects that are to be addressed. The Amplatzer Septal Occluder has the advantage of being applicable to a wide range of defect diameters but, therefore, requires a large stock (sizes 4 to 20 mm in 1-mm increments; sizes 22 to 40 in 2-mm increments). The most commonly used implant for muscular ventricular septal defects is that designed by AGA Medical, the Amplatzer Septal Occluder. It is easy to deliver to the target lesion, retrievable, and comes in several sizes (4- through 18-mm diameter central plugs). These devices also can be used for other occlusions (eg, atrial implants can be used in ventricular defects, in persistently patent arterial ducts, or in fistulas).

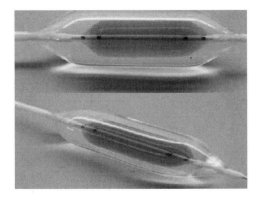

Fig. 5. The BIB balloon has an inner balloon, constructed from the same material as the so-called "Tyshak II" balloon, whereas the outer balloon is constructed from a heavier gauge material as used in the Z-Med higher pressure balloon. The BIB balloon allows controlled delivery of stents and adjustment of stent position after inflation of the inner balloon. This prevents stent migration and the balloon design prevents flaring of the stent.

*Endovascular stents*

There are several endovascular stents that are useful in interventional management of patients who have a congenital heart lesion. Operators should be familiar with one or two types, noting their advantages and limitations. In the adult setting, stocking a range of sizes and lengths can be rationalized, particularly for use in aortic coarctation. In this case, it seems that a covered stent (see later discussion) is the safest form of implant. There are several choices, including but not limited to the Palmaz Genesis or XL (Johnson & Johnson, Warren, New Jersey), Cheatham-Platinum (CP) (NuMed), Jomed (Jomed NV), Wallstent (Boston Scientific), Corinthian (Johnson & Johnson). There is a limited number of covered stents applicable to adults who have congenital heart lesions, primarily because of available expansion ratios (eg, Jomed, Gore, Medtronic, Wallstent, and CP stents).

In addition to their use in aortic coarctation, they have an important role as standby or bailout. The CP stent is the covered stent used most commonly for congenital lesions. It is made of platinum and iridium, with gold used to strengthen the 0.013-inch–thick wire solders. Unlike other implants, they have rounded leading and trailing edges that reduce the risk of balloon rupture during inflation and of vessel trauma. Its visibility is good; it can be expanded to large diameters (up to 25 mm); and delivery can be through 12-Fr sheaths. Importantly, the implant is MRI compatible, a significant issue when managing adults (Fig. 8).

In summary, careful thought in stocking a laboratory with a wide variety of equipment for all types of interventional procedures is required for

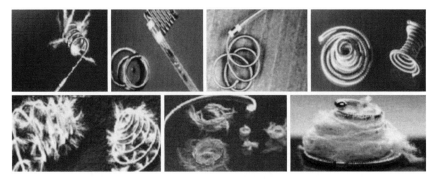

Fig. 6. The top three panels from the left depict controlled release implants; the remaining panels show a few of the many shapes that can be useful in particular locations.

an effective program. Although considerable variations in kinds of equipment are required, a rational inventory with a focus on adult applications easily is achievable and at a reasonable expense.

## Flows and shunts

### The sample run

In the decision-making process for patients who have a congenital heart lesion, a great deal of significance is placed on oxygen saturation data. As an isolated measurement, the determination of blood oxygen saturation can provide important information about patients early in the catheterization procedure. Arterial desaturation may reflect a right-to-left shunt or a ventilation-perfusion mismatch. Systemic venous saturation less than

50% indicates a low cardiac output; a high saturation indicates either a left-to-right shunt or high output state. The calculation of cardiac outputs, shunts, and resistances is dependent on an accurate determination of oxygen saturation. There are several assumptions in using oxygen as an indicator (see later discussion), however, and some practical considerations in obtaining oxygen saturation data, and potential errors can be introduced. As such, oxygen saturation data is the least sensitive and most prone to error of all the physiologic data obtained in a catheter laboratory.

Assumptions when using oxygen as an indicator are:

All measurements are made during steady-state blood flow. In other words, there are

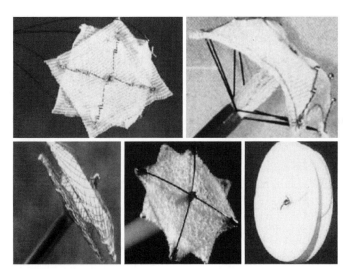

Fig. 7. A few of the available atrial defect implants are shown. Top panels: the CardioSEAL (*left*) and Starflex (*right*). In the lower panel, the Amplatzer Septal Occluder (*left*), Cardia (*middle*), and Helex (*right*).

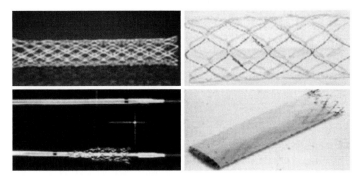

Fig. 8. Various stents are available. As an example, the Genesis balloon expandable stent is seen in the left upper panel, and a self-expanding Wallstent in the left lower panel. The bare metal and covered CP stent are shown in the right upper and lower panels, respectively.

no changes in blood flow, respiratory rate, heart rate, or level of consciousness.

Two or more samples are obtained from at least three sites in rapid succession, which, in patients who have complex congenital heart disorders, can be difficult to achieve. For flow determinations (not discussed in this article), the assumption is that the samples are taken at the same time that oxygen consumption is measured.

*The mixed venous saturation*

There is no single uniform source for mixed venous blood, as the "mixed" venous blood sample has three variable sources, that is, the inferior vena cava (IVC), the coronary sinus, and the superior vena cava (SVC), with each caval vein having multiple sources of blood with different saturations.

The SVC oxygen saturation may vary by 10%, as it receives blood from the jugular, subclavian, and azygous systems, each with different saturations and flows (the subclavian and azygous veins have higher saturations than the jugular vein). The IVC also has variable oxygen saturations, as the components that make up its flow may vary by up to 10% to 20%. For example, more saturated blood originates from the renal veins, whereas less saturated blood comes from gastrocolic and hepatic sources. The net mixed sample from the IVC generally is 5% to 10% greater then the SVC. Coronary sinus blood also contributes to the total pool of mixed systemic return. Despite making up only 5% to 7% of total venous return, the very low saturation in this sample (25%–45%) can have an impact on the total mixed saturation.

As there are multiple contributions to the so-called "mixed" venous sample, there is no practical way to measure each and account for the variations in flow. Not even a sample from the right atrium can adjust for streaming completely. In the absence of a shunt lesion, a sample downstream from the right atrium, such as from the main pulmonary artery, can provide for a thoroughly "mixed" sample. Also, it has been noted that the SVC blood saturation is close to that in the main pulmonary artery and can be used as representative of the mixed venous sample unless patients have a low cardiac output state. Some investigators use a weighted average of SVC and IVC blood (see later discussion) as a calculated mixed venous sample. In the presence of a downstream shunt lesion, several samples, obtained in rapid sequence and found to be near or equal in value, should be used.

Similarly, the mixed pulmonary venous saturation is a combination of all the pulmonary veins, each reflecting different ventilation-to-perfusion ratios. As such, a pulmonary vein sample may be 50% to 100% disparate from the "true" mixed venous sample. In the absence of a right-to-left shunt, a downstream sample is preferable (left ventricle or aorta) to using a single pulmonary vein saturation. In the presence of a right-to-left shunt, the assumptions are even more difficult. If there is a distal right-to-left shunt, then the most distal left atrial sample, at the orifice of the mitral valve, should be used.

*Sampling*

When blood is drawn for shunt calculations, the samples should be obtained proximally and distally to the lesion. Note must be taken of the influence of streaming, where a saturation gradient may exist. Samples must be drawn in rapid temporal sequence, no more than 1 to 2 minutes for the sampling run. Duplicate samples should be obtained when possible and should differ by no more then 1% or 2%. Operators must be aware of potential equipment malfunctions as a source of differing sample values. When a sample is drawn, all flush solution and blood must be cleared from the catheter and the catheter filled with the sample blood by a further withdraw. If there is a poor connection between the catheter and syringe or significant negative pressure is applied, then microbubbles can be drawn into the sample, resulting in oxygenation. Samples should not be drawn from the side arm of a bleed-back tap, as they contain a chamber where the sample can be contaminated. This also applies to stopcock valves, where a small amount of blood remains in the connecting chamber and contaminates the sample.

*Clinical applications*

In patients who have congenital heart disease in whom a communication between the two sides of the heart, or between the aorta and the pulmonary artery, allows a shunt to exist, several calculations may be made, namely: (1) the magnitude of a left-to-right shunt, (2) the magnitude of a right-to-left shunt, (3) effective pulmonary blood flow (PBF), and (4) pulmonary-to-systemic-blood-flow ratio (Qp:Qs).

Of these, the only calculation that is of practical value is Qp:Qs. This provides a simple and reliable estimate of the extent to which PBF is increased or reduced and provides a useful insight into the severity of the hemodynamic disturbance in most cases. It also is simple to perform, using solely the oxygen saturation data from systemic arterial blood, left atrial/pulmonary venous blood, pulmonary artery, and vena caval/right heart samples.

The samples need to be acquired in (or be ventilated with) room air or a gas mixture containing no more than a maximum of 30% oxygen. If oxygen-enriched gas (>30% oxygen) is being given, the saturation data may not provide accurate information regarding PBF, as a significant amount of oxygen may be present in dissolved form in the pulmonary venous sample (which is not factored into the calculation if saturations alone are used). Under such circumstances, pulmonary flow tends to be overestimated and the Qp:Qs exaggerated correspondingly.

*The pulmonary-to-systemic-blood-flow ratio*

This calculation is based on the Fick principle; that is, factors, such as oxygen-carrying capacity and oxygen consumption, that are used for individual calculations (for pulmonary and systemic flows) cancel out when only the ratio of the two flows is estimated. This is convenient as it removes the more difficult and time-consuming parts of the calculation. The resulting equation (after removing the factors that cancel out) is pleasingly simple: Qp:Qs = (Sat Ao−Sat MV)/(Sat PV−Sat PA), where Sat Ao is aortic saturation, Sat MV is mixed venous saturation, Sat PV is pulmonary vein saturation, and Sat PA is pulmonary artery saturation.

As the aortic saturation and pulmonary artery saturation are measured routinely, the only components that may present any problem are the pulmonary vein saturation and the mixed venous saturation (see previous discussion). If a pulmonary vein has not been entered, an assumed value of 98% may be used (note the potential error). The left atrial saturation can be substituted provided there is no right-to-left shunt at atrial level. Similarly, left ventricular or aortic saturation may be substituted, provided there is no right-to-left shunt. For mixed venous saturation, the tradition is to use the most distal right heart location if there is no left-to-right shunt. Thus, the pulmonary artery sample should be used if there is no shunt at atrial or ventricular level.

In practice, the SVC saturation often is used, although some prefer to use a value intermediate between the SVC and IVC (see previous discussion). It has been demonstrated, however, that the mixed venous saturation approximates the SVC more closely than the IVC. The following formula often is used: mixed venous saturation (MV) = (3 times the Sat SVC + the Sat IVC)/4. A simple way of calculating this ("in your head") is to use the formula, MV = Sat SVC−(Sat SVC−Sat IVC)/4. Thus, if SVC saturation is 78% and IVC saturation is 70%, MV should be 76% (78−70 = 8; 8/4 = 2; 78−2 = 76).

*The usefulness of the shunt ratio in practice*

The Qp:Qs is useful, for instance, in making decisions about surgery for patients who have a ventricular defect. Beyond infancy, a Qp:Qs greater than 1.8:1 likely requires intervention, whereas less than 1.5:1 does not. Qp:Qs also is helpful in assessing the hemodynamics of many more complex defects, but it should be recognized that under some circumstances it is of limited practical help. In atrial defects, if there is evidence of a significant shunt on clinical and noninvasive testing (right ventricular dilatation, paradoxic septal motion, cardiomegaly on radiograph, or right ventricular hypertrophy on ECG), the shunt ratio should not be used to decide about treatment. This is because atrial shunts depend on right ventricular filling characteristics, which can vary depending on conditions (sympathetic tone or catecholamine concentrations). It is not uncommon for a measured shunt to be small (for example, <1.5:1) despite other evidence of a significant defect.

### Coronary arteriography

This section does not attempt to discuss all anomalies of the coronary circulation in any detail, as excellent reviews may be found in the literature [1,2]. Instead it focuses on the more common anomalies faced by adult congenital angiographers and some possible approaches to consider. First, it is useful to consider a working classification of the type of coronary anomalies seen in structurally normal and abnormal hearts. Freedom and Culham [3] present an excellent review of these anomalies and divide the possibilities into four groups as outlined in Box 1.

For adult angiographers, one of the more common and often frustrating presentations is "the missing coronary artery." A frequent mistake is to assume that the origin of the artery is indeed in its expected position in or just above the midpoint of its facing sinus. An operator then may persist for inordinate lengths of time with the usual Judkins-shape catheter, believing the vessel is there and that further catheter manipulation will identify its origin. If the usual shape catheter does not identify the origin quickly, consider the alternatives. Coronary arteries may connect to the aorta immediately adjacent to a commissure, to the ascending aorta well above the sinotubular junction, or to the contralateral facing sinus. In addition, the coronary circulation may have a single main coronary artery, with the right coronary, circumflex, and left anterior descending arteries all arising from the trunk, with the main trunk itself having an anomalous aortic wall or sinus origin. Similarly, it is not uncommon to find an individual artery arising from another coronary artery, for example the circumflex or left anterior descending artery from the right coronary, or the right coronary from the left coronary artery. If the left coronary artery cannot be found

**Box 1. Classification of coronary artery anomalies**

1. Anomalies of origin
   A. Ostial anomalies
   B. Ectopic origin
      i. Anomalous origin from the aortic wall or sinus
      ii. Anomalous origin from a coronary artery
      iii. Abnormal connection to a pulmonary artery
      iv. Origin from a vessel other than the pulmonary artery or aorta
      v. Origin from a ventricular cavity

2. Anomalies of course
   A. Intramural course
   B. Aberrant course of proximal coronary artery
   C. Myocardial bridge
   D. Epicardial crossing

3. Anomalies of termination or connection
   A. Connections to cardiac structures
   B. Connections to extracardiac structures

4. Anomalies of coronary size

with the left Judkins catheter in the left coronary sinus, or if the circumflex or left anterior descending is "missing," the next step is to proceed to the right coronary artery, which usually identifies the missing artery arising from the right coronary trunk. If the right coronary artery is the missing artery, then an aortogram or review of the left ventricular angiogram often identifies the anomalous origin. The operator then must select from the variety of catheter shapes available the best fit for the location in the aortic wall of the origin. Although there are no hard and fast rules, often the Amplatzer shapes and multipurpose catheter are first choices to reach anomalous origins.

When a proximal coronary artery, in particular the circumflex or left anterior descending, has an aberrant course from the anterior facing sinus, it is important to define which of four courses the vessel pursues to reach the left ventricle: retroaortic, interarterial, right ventricular free wall, or infundibular septum. Some criteria are available and, combined with careful angiography, help make the correct diagnosis [4,5]. This becomes important if a cardiac surgical procedure is planned.

The other not infrequent finding that arises for adult congenital angiographers is one or more coronary arteriovenous fistulae. These may connect from either coronary artery, be quite small or very large, be single or multiple, and connect to a chamber, usually right-sided, or to a coronary vein or coronary sinus. Most are small, exit in a mediastinal vessel, do not require any intervention, and are of passing interest. A few are large and associated with symptoms or signs of volume overload and lead to the question of catheter or surgical intervention. In these few cases, angiographers should spend the time and make additional contrast injections in multiple projections to define the exact origin of the fistula carefully and the anatomy of the exit of the fistula. These are important in deciding if catheter occlusion is possible, if surgery is necessary, and the best interventional or surgical approach to closure.

## Chamber angiography

Accurate anatomic and physiologic diagnosis is the foundation of a successful catheter-based therapeutic procedure. This section includes a discussion of standard angiographic approaches and how to achieve them. Emphasis is placed on the application of these projections as applied to interventional procedures. A detailed description of the physical principles of image formation is beyond the scope of this article and interested readers are referred to other sources for more detailed information [6].

### Angiographic projections

In the therapeutic management of patients who have a congenital heart lesion, the spatial orientation and detailed morphology of the heart and great vessels are of critical importance (Table 1). As an operator enters a laboratory, an understanding of the anatomy should have been synthesized, based on information from other imaging modalities, such as chest roentgenography, echocardiography, CT, and MRI. As such, the angiographic projections used in the procedure are tailored to outline the lesion to allow appropriate measurements and guide the intervention.

The heart is oriented obliquely, with the left ventricular apex leftward, anterior, and inferior, in relation to the base of the heart. The interventricular septum is a complex geometric

Table 1
Angiographic projections

| Projection | Angles |
| --- | --- |
| Single plane projections | |
| Conventional RAO | 40° RAO |
| Frontal | 0° |
| Shallow LAO | 1° to 30° |
| Straight LAO | 31° to 60° |
| Steep LAO | 61° to 89° |
| Left lateral | 90° left |
| Cranially tilted RAO | 30° RAO + 30° cranial |
| Cranially tilted frontal (sitting-up view) | 30° or 45° cranial |
| Cranially tilted shallow LAO | 25° LAO + 30° cranial |
| Cranially tilted mid LAO (long axis oblique) | 60° LAO + 20°–30° cranial |
| Cranially tilted steep LAO (hepatoclavicular view) | 45° to 70° LAO + 30° cranial |
| Caudally tilted frontal | 45° caudal |

| Biplane combinations | A plane | B plane |
| --- | --- | --- |
| AP and LAT | 0° | Left lateral |
| Long axial oblique | 30° RAO | 60° LAO + 20° to 30° cranial |
| Hepatoclavicular view | 45° LAO + 30° cranial | 120° LAO + 15° cranial |
| Specific lesions | | |
| RVOT-MPA (sitting up) | 10° LAO + 40° cranial | Left lateral |
| Long axial for LPA (biplane) | 30° RAO | 60° LAO + 30° cranial |
| LPA long axis (single plane) | | 60° LAO + 20° cranial |
| ASD | 30° LAO + 30° cranial | |
| PA bifurcation and branches | 30° caudal + 10° 20° caudal RAO | |

Primary projections are in italics.
*Abbreviations:* LPA, left pulmonary artery; MPA, main pulmonary artery; RVOT, right ventricular outflow tract; PA, pulmonary artery.

3-D structure that takes an S-curve from apex to base, the so-called "sigmoid septum." From caudal to cranial, the interventricular septum curves through an arc of 100° to 120°, and the right ventricle appears as an appliqué or overlay on the left ventricle. To address this topology, today's angiographic equipment allows a wide range of projections, incorporating caudocranial or craniocaudal angulations. The up-to-date laboratory consists of independent biplane imaging chains, which, with the proper selection of views, minimizes overlapping and foreshortening of structures.

*Terminology*

Angiographic projections are designated either according to the position of the recording detector (image intensifier or flat panel detector) or the direction of the x-ray beam toward the recording device. In cardiology, the convention usually is the former. For example, when the detector is directly above a supine patient, the x-ray beam travels from posterior to anterior and the angiographic projection is designated posteroanterior (PA), but based on detector position, it is called frontal, and the position of the detector by convention is at 0°. Similarly, when the detector is moved through 90°, to a position beside and to the left of a patient, a lateral (LAT) projection results. Between 0° and 90°, there are a multitude of projections, termed left anterior oblique (LAO), and when the detector is moved to the right of a patient, a right anterior oblique (RAO) projection is achieved. Standard detectors mounted on a C-arm or parallelogram not only allow these positions but also the detectors can be rotated around the transverse axis, toward the feet or head, caudally or cranially (Fig. 9).

*Biplane angiography*

A dedicated interventional catheterization laboratory addressing congenital heart defects requires biplane facilities [7,8]. Biplane angiography has the advantage of limiting contrast exposure and evaluating the cardiac structures in real-time in two projections simultaneously. This is at a cost, however, as these facilities are expensive,

and with existing image intensifiers and newer flat panel detectors, extreme simultaneous angulations can be compromised. Standard biplane configurations include RAO/LAO and frontal/lateral projections, with additional cranial or caudal tilt. The possible combinations are endless (see Box 1; see Fig. 1).

*Cranial–left anterior oblique projections*

A clear working understanding of these projections is of critical importance in developing a flexible approach to congenital heart defect angiography and intervention. The practice of using "cookbook" projections for each case may allow acceptable diagnostic studies but falls short of the detail required to accomplish an interventional procedure. A comprehensive understanding of normal cardiac anatomy, especially the interventricular septum, allows operators to adjust the projection to profile the region of interest optimally.

There are several rules of thumb that allow operators to judge the steepness or shallowness of an LAO projection. Of importance is the relationship of the cardiac silhouette to the spine, the ventricular catheter, and the ventricular apex.

To optimize the profile of the midpoint of the membranous ventricular septum (thus, the majority of perimembranous defects), two thirds of the cardiac silhouette should be to the right of the vertebral bodies (Figs. 10 and 11). This results in a cranially tilted left ventriculogram showing the left ventricular septal wall, with the apex (denoted by the ventricular catheter) pointing toward the bottom of the image. A shallower projection has more of the cardiac silhouette over toward the left of the spine and profiles the inferobasal component of the septum, ideal for inlet type ventricular defects. This projection allows for evaluation of atrioventricular valve relationships, inlet extension of perimembranous defects, and posterior

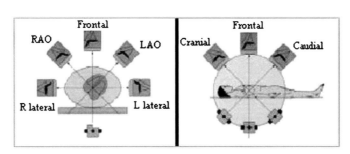

Fig. 9. Angiographic projections in biplane. L, left; R, right.

542 MCLAUGHLIN et al

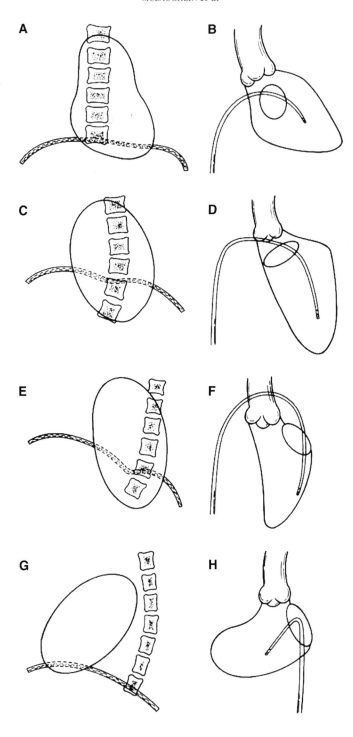

muscular defects. A steeper LAO projection can be used to profile the outlet extension of a perimembranous defect and anterior muscular and apical defects. As noted in Fig. 10, the ventricular catheter in the cardiac apex can be used to help guide the projection, but only if it enters the chamber through the mitral valve. If catheter entry is through the ventricular defect or retrograde, it tends to be more basal and left lateral.

Modification of the cranial LAO projection has to be made if there is a discrepancy in chamber sizes, and the septum is rotated such that a steeper or shallower projection may be required. Also, it is assumed that a patient is lying flat on the examining table, but if the head is turned to the right or there is a pad under the buttocks, it rotates the thorax such that the LAO projection is steeper and the detector caudal. This has to be compensated for during the set-up for the angiogram. The clue in the former case is that the more of the heart silhouette is over the spine.

The first step in setting up a cranial-LAO projection is to achieve the correct degree of steepness or shallowness. After that, the degree of cranial tilt has to be confirmed, so that the basal-apical septum is elongated. This can be estimated by seeing how much of the hemidiaphragm is superimposed over the cardiac silhouette; the greater the superimposition, the greater the cranial tilt. Additionally, the degree of cranial tilt can be determined by looking at the course of the ventricular catheter, which appears to be foreshortened or coming directly at the viewer as the degree of cranial angulation is decreased (Fig. 12).

## Specific lesions

### Ventricular septal defect

The imaging of specific ventricular defects (Fig. 13) is beyond the scope of this review but is commented on in detail by various investigators

[9]. The injections to outline the septum and the margins that circumscribe the defects are performed best in the left ventricle using a power injector. Two orthogonal (right-angle) projections give the best chance of profiling the lesion. Table 1 lists single and biplane angulations for the various projections. For the perimembranous defect, the midcranial LAO projection, at approximately 50° to 60° LAO, and as much cranial tilt as the equipment and patient position allow (see Fig. 10) should be attempted. Additional projections can include a shallow LAO with cranial tilt (so-called "four-chamber" or hepatoclavicular view) to outline the basal septum or inlet extension of a perimembranous defect. The RAO view outlines the high anterior and infundibular (outlet) defects [10].

### Coarctation of the aorta

Biplane angiography should be used to outline the aortic arch lesion (Fig. 14). Projections that can be used include LAO/RAO, frontal and LAT, or a shallow or steep LAO. The authors' preference is a 30° LAO and left LAT, with 10° to 15° caudal tilt to minimize any overlapping structures, such as a ductal bump or diverticulum. Modifications to accommodate a right arch generally are mirror-image projections (ie, 30° RAO and left LAT). Operators must be cautious to examine the transverse arch for associated hypoplasia, and this may be foreshortened in the straight left-LAT projection. In such an instance, for a left arch, a left posterior oblique projection may elongate the arch. This is important particularly if an endovascular stent is deployed near the head and neck vessels.

### Aortic valve angiography

In the setting of normally related great arteries with ventriculoarterial concordance, assessment of the diameter of the aortic valve for balloon dilation is performed best using biplane in the long

---

Fig. 10. Setting up a standard LAO projection. To achieve the LAO projection, attempt to adjust the detector angle so that two thirds of the cardiac silhouette is to the left of the spine as in (E). If a catheter is through the mitral valve in the left ventricular apex, it points to the floor, as in (F). In this view, the intraventricular septal margin points toward the floor. The so-called "4-chamber" or hepatoclavicular view is achieved by having half the cardiac silhouette over the spine, as in (C). A catheter across the mitral valve appears as in (D). A steep LAO projection has the cardiac silhouette as in (G), and a transmitral catheter in the left ventricle appears as in (H). (A) and (B) show the frontal projection. (*Modified from* Culham JAG. Physical principles of image formation and projections in angiocardiography. In: Freedom RM, Mawson JB, Yoo SJ, et al, editors. Congenital heart disease textbook of angiocardiography. Armonk, NY: Futura Publishing; 1997. p. 9–93; with permission.)

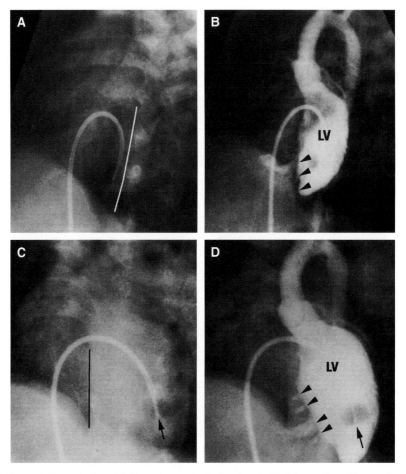

Fig. 11. Achieving an LAO projection. (*A*) For a hepatoclavicular view, half of the cardiac silhouette is over or just left of the spine, with the catheter pointing toward the left of the image. During the injection, the apex and catheter (*arrow*) point toward the bottom and left of the image. In this example, the basal (inlet) portion of the septum in intact. In (*B*) multiple midmuscular septal defects are not well profiled (*arrowheads*). In (*C*), the LAO projection is achieved with the catheter pointing toward the bottom (*arrow*) of the frame and the cardiac silhouette well over the spine. During the contrast injection (*D*), the midmuscular defects (*arrow*) are profiled better. (*Modified from* Culham JAG. Physical principles of image formation and projections in angiocardiography. In: Freedom RM, Mawson JB, Yoo SJ, et al, editors. Congenital heart disease textbook of angiocardiography. Armonk, NY: Futura Publishing; 1997. p. 39–93; with permission.)

axis and RAO projections (Fig. 15; see Table 1). The authors' preference is to obtain the diameter of the aortic valve from a ventriculogram, which profiles the hinge points of the leaflets. Caution must be observed when using an ascending aortogram, as one of the leaflets of the valve may obscure the margins of attachment.

*The Mustard baffle*

Over time, patients who have had a Mustard operation may develop obstruction to one or both limbs of the venous baffle (Fig. 16). As atrial arrhythmias are not uncommon in such adult patients, pacing systems frequently are required for management. To facilitate pacing catheter insertion, enlargement of a stenotic, often asymptomatic, superior baffle frequently is required. The optimum projection to outline superior baffle obstruction for potential stent implantation is a cranially angulated LAO projection (30° LAO and 30° cranial). This view elongates the baffle pathway, allowing accurate measurement before stenting. For inferior baffle lesions, a frontal projection allows adequate localization of the lesion. Leaks along the baffle are more problematic and require

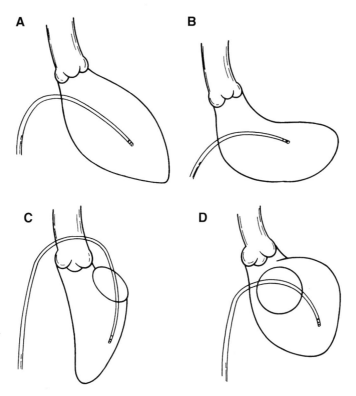

Fig. 12. Obtaining the cranial tilt. In the standard RAO view (*A*), the left ventricular apex points caudally and to the left. The LAO view opens the outflow from apex to base, as in diagram (*C*). If there is an upturned apex as in Fallot's tetralogy the RAO view appears as in (*B*). Adding cranial tilt to a mid-LAO projection does not open the apex to base projection effectively, and the appearance is as looking down the barrel of the ventricles, as in (*D*). (*Modified from* Culham JAG. Physical principles of image formation and projections in angiocardiography. In: Freedom RM, Mawson JB, Yoo SJ, et al, editors. Congenital heart disease textbook of angiocardiography. Armonk, NY: Futura Publishing; 1997. p. 39–93; with permission.)

modification of the projection. The initial approach should be a frontal projection, with modifications in angulation made thereafter to best profile the lesion for device implantation.

*The secundum atrial septal defect and the fenestrated Fontan*

Secundum ASDs are profiled best in the 30° LAO with 30° cranial tilt (Figs. 17 and 18). With the injection made in the right upper pulmonary vein, the sinus venosus portion of the septum can be visualized, and anomalous pulmonary venous return ruled out. Additionally, any associated septal aneurysm can be outlined. With the application of transesophageal echocardiography (TEE) or intracardiac echocardiography, there is less reliance on fluoroscopic device positioning. When balloon sizing is performed, this projection elongates the axis of the balloon for proper measurements.

The interventional management of patients who have a fenestrated Fontan, either a lateral tunnel or extracardiac connection, generally requires selective studies of the SVC and IVC and pulmonary circulations to determine the presence or absence of obstructive or hypoplastic pathways and whether or not venous collaterals have developed. If present, they must be addressed by angioplasty, stenting, or embolization techniques before fenestration closure. Venous collaterals after an extracardiac Fontan generally develop either from the innominate vein or from the right upper hepatic/phrenic vein, toward the neoleft atrium, less frequently from the right hepatic veins to the pulmonary veins. The optimum projection to outline these lesions is in the frontal and LAT projections, with selective power injections in the

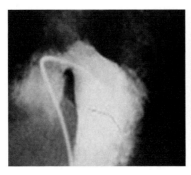
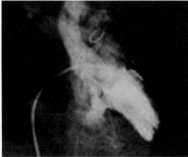

Fig. 13. (*Left*) Long axis oblique projection of a left ventriculogram, defining a perimembranous ventricular septal defect. (*Right*) A midmuscular defect outlined with a hepatoclavicular left ventricular injection.

appropriate vessel. The location and dimensions of the fenestration also may be defined in these views, but for ideal profiling, some degree of right or left anterior obliquity may be required.

*The bidirectional cavopulmonary connection*

Second-stage palliation for several congenital defects consists of a bidirectional cavopulmonary connection (also known as the bidirectional Glenn anastomosis). Because the caval to pulmonary artery connection is toward the anterior surface of the right pulmonary artery (rather than on the upper surface), an anteroposterior (AP) projection results in overlapping of the anastomotic site with the pulmonary artery. Therefore, to determine whether or not the anastomosis is obstructed, a 30° caudal with 10° LAO projection generally opens that region for better definition (Fig. 19).

Furthermore, this projection outlines the full extent of the right and left pulmonary arteries. The left-LAT projection, with or without 10° caudal angulation, profiles the anastomosis for its anterior-posterior dimension. Contrast injection must be made in the lower portion of the SVC. Examination of venous collaterals can be performed from the AP and LAT projections in the innominate vein.

*Pulmonary valve stenosis and Fallot's tetralogy*

Percutaneous intervention on isolated pulmonary valve stenosis was the procedure that ushered in the current era of catheter-based therapies (Fig. 20). Although angiographic definition of the right ventricular outflow tract and valve is not complicated, several features must be kept in mind when approaching angiography for an

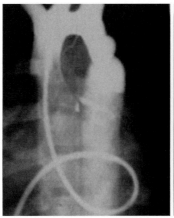
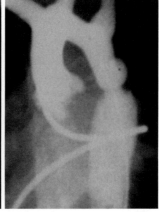

Fig. 14. Left panel shows an ascending aortogram taken with a shallow-LAO projection without caudal angulation. The catheter was placed through a transeptal entry to the left heart. Although the area of the coarctation can be seen, it is the caudal angulation that identifies the details of the lesion, including a small ductal ampulla (*right panel*).

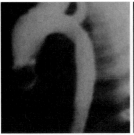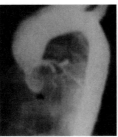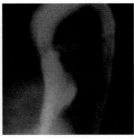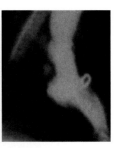

Fig. 15. Intervention on the aortic valve requires accurate definition of the hinge points of the leaflets. In the two left panels, long axis oblique views from an ascending aortogram, the margins of the leaflets are not defined because of overlap of the cusps (bicuspid in these examples). In the two right panels, long axis oblique (*left*) and RAO views, the left ventriculogram allows easier identification of the leaflet hinge points, where measurements can be made.

interventional procedure. In the case of isolated pulmonary valve stenosis and other right ventricular outflow tract lesions, because the outflow tract can take a horizontal curve, a simple AP projection foreshortens the structure. Therefore, a 30° cranial with 15° LAO opens up the infundibulum, allowing visualization of the valve and the main and branch pulmonary arteries. The best definition of the hinge points of the valve, to choose the correct balloon size, is from the left-LAT projection. Occasionally, 10° or 15° caudal angulation of the LAT detector can be used to separate the overlap of the branch vessels seen on a straight left-LAT projection. This is not recommended, however, as it also foreshortens the outflow tract and the valve appears off plane, giving incorrect valve diameters.

*Branch pulmonary artery stenosis*

Pulmonary artery interventions are common and represent the most difficult angiographic projections to separate out individual vessels for assessment and potential intervention (Figs. 21 and 22). A cranially tilted frontal projection with left-LAT or RAO/LAO projections frequently is the first series of views that can be performed as scout studies to map the proximal and hilar regions of the pulmonary circulation. The injection may be performed either in the ventricle or main pulmonary artery. Because there is frequent overlap in viewing the right ventricular outflow tract (see previous discussion), these standard views can be modified by increasing or decreasing the degree of RAO or LAO and adding caudal or cranial tilt. Selective branch artery injections are best for detailed visualization to plan the intervention. For the right pulmonary artery, a shallow RAO projection with 10° or 15° cranial tilt

separates the upper and middle lobe branches, whereas a left LAT with 15° caudal tilt opens up all the anterior vessels. Similarly, to maximize the elongated and posterior leftward directed left pulmonary artery, a 60° LAO with 20° cranial is effective, with a caudal tilt on the lateral detector.

## The changing indications for cardiac catheterization in adult congential heart disease

There has been no greater impact on the care of patients who have congenital heart disease than the new imaging modalities. The heart, once accessible only by surgeons, angiocardiographers, and pathologists, now can be sliced safely and accurately, rotated, and examined with minimal discomfort to patients. The development of better imaging has had a great impact on the ability to make decisions and plan percutaneous interventions and surgery.

Unfortunately, the clinical appreciation of patient anatomy can become quite befuddled as years go by and patients are cared for by different pediatricians and adult cardiologists or even lost to specialized follow-up. This is never so true as when geographic migrations occur and patients leave a pediatric hospital where they were cared for initially and arrive in a new city without their medical file.

Clinical information about patients has a hierarchy in terms of relevance and importance. A tattered 25-year-old surgical report may be the Holy Grail of information. A seasoned surgeon's operative report may describe carefully native and surgical anatomy in great detail. The report may provide insight into what was repaired and how and why. A close second in the hierarchy is a good-quality CT scan or MRI by an experienced

548     MCLAUGHLIN et al

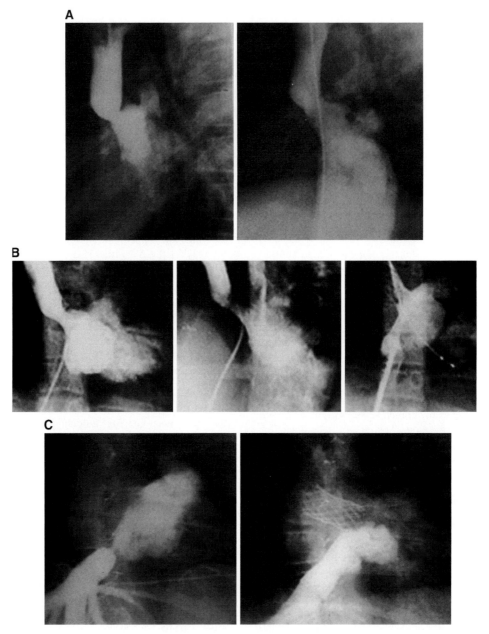

Fig. 16. Baffle obstruction after a Mustard operation is, as the population ages, an increasingly common event. This is important particularly when such patients need transvenous pacing devices. In (*A*) (*left panel*), the presence of a superior baffle obstruction can be identified from the left LAT projection. Only with cranial angulation (cranial-LAO view) (*right panel*), however, is the full extent of the lesion detailed. This is critical (*B*), particularly where the frontal view (*left panel*), does not show the full extent of the obstruction, and only from the angulated view are the length and diameter of the lesion outlined (*middle panel*). A stent is placed, followed by a transvenous pacing system, as shown in the right panel from a frontal projection. For an inferior baffle lesion, the frontal (PA) projection is optimal (*C*), before (*left*) and after (*right*) a stent is placed.

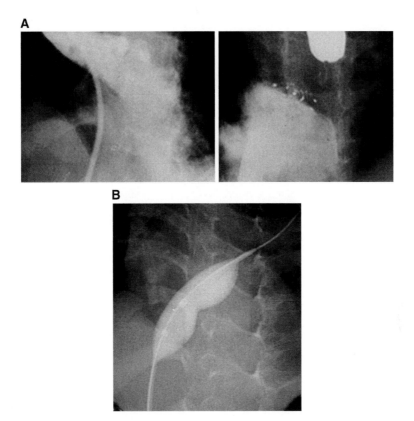

Fig. 17. Use of angiography for septal defect definition and device placement in the setting of a secundum ASD has been supplanted by intracardiac and transesophageal techniques (*A*). Fluoroscopy still is required for initial device localization, however, and in many laboratories, a short cine-run to record the diameter of the static balloon diameter to choose device size. In this case, the authors find the 30° LAO with 30° cranial tilt to best elongate the balloon to avoid foreshortening (*B*).

imager. The latest generation of imaging equipment from the major modalities of echo, MRI, and CT permits the appreciation of the most subtle anatomic detail.

More important than the newest technology and costliest equipment is the availability of imaging specialists to conduct the study, interpret it expertly, report it insightfully, and caution if there are limitations that should be known about. Collaboration between image and clinical, surgical, and interventional physicians allows the integration of knowledge and facilitates the delivery of excellent patient care. Little is gained from the ability to produce beautiful images that are interpreted in a way that is not meaningful to clinicians. It is as important for radiologists to know the concerns of surgeons and interventionalists as is the reverse. Choosing the right modality to answer a particular question or set of questions is key, as is providing imagers with the specific questions to be

addressed so that correct protocols are used to obtain the information required.

*Echocardiography*

Echocardiography always will play an important role in the care of patients who have ACHD. Its availability, portability, and familiarity to most recently trained cardiologists is a strength. Echocardiographers trained to interpret complex anatomy in congenital heart disease are a necessity. The ability to assess patients rapidly at the bedside in an emergency department, during off hours, and in an ICU is a definite benefit, especially when patients are critically ill. Echo provides important structural and physiologic information and is the noninvasive reference standard for valvular assessment. TEE or, more recently, intracardiac echocardiography is helpful especially during interventional procedures. These

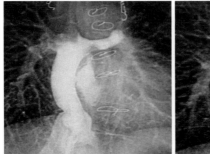
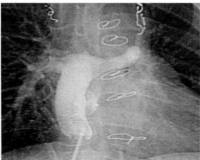

Fig. 18. Left panel shows the appearance of a fenestrated extracardiac Fontan in the frontal projection, the right panel its appearance after device closure. Generally, a frontal projection profiles the defect adequately, but at times some angulation is required, where the defect is profiled best in a shallow RAO view. Also, note coils in the left SVC, which developed after the Fontan procedure and required embolization. Occasionally, collateral vessels develop from the hepatic/phrenic vein or innominate vein, the primary view being frontal and left LAT.

modalities allow the real-time monitoring and detailed evaluation of device implantation or valvular intervention in an unobtrusive and minimally limiting fashion.

*Cross-sectional imaging*

MRI and CT are critical imaging modalities for clinicians. MRI provides tremendous anatomic detail and functional information. Gradients across valvular orifices, planimetry of valve areas, relative pulmonary flow, and collateral vessel flow are in the repertoire of experienced imagers. Hints are provided to the presence of small ASDs or baffle leaks. The ability to postprocess a data set adds to its versatility and permits post hoc evaluation of new questions immediately or years

in the future. The examinations are lengthy and require significant time to reconstruct the data. MRI, however, lacks global applicability to all patients. Patients who have pacing devices or similar implants, cerebral aneurysm clips, or foreign bodies in an eye may not be studied at this time. Patients who have nonplatinum coils, stents, or devices may be imaged but are not well suited to this investigation. The artifact caused by many devices distorts the magnetic field and renders the area of interest inaccessible. As the examinations are lengthy and many MRI bores still are closed, narrow, and dark, it is not uncommon for patients to be unable to tolerate an examination for reasons of discomfort or claustrophobia. It is possible to prepare patients properly with information or medication to overcome this problem but if

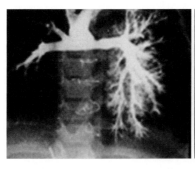
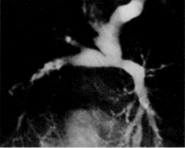

Fig. 19. Because of an offset in the anastomosis between the SVC and right pulmonary artery, the optimal view to see the anastomosis without overlap is a shallow one—with caudal tilt as seen in the right panel. In the left panel, in the frontal projection, there is overlap of the anastomosis which obscures a potential lesion, as seen in the angulated view. The combination of an angulated frontal detector and caudal angulation of the lateral tube allows definition of the anastomosis and the pulmonary artery confluence.

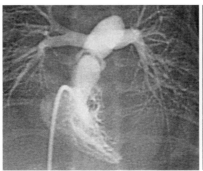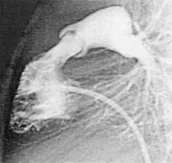

Fig. 20. Left panel depicts a case of typical isolated pulmonary valve stenosis in a neonate. The outflow tract is profiled in the cranially angulated frontal projection, with a slight degree of LAO angulation. The right ventriculogram outlines the form of the ventricle, the main pulmonary artery (and ductal bump), and the pulmonary artery confluence and branch dimensions. The LAT view (*right panel*) outlines the valve leaflets (thickened and doming) and allows accurate delineation of the valve structures for balloon diameter determination.

unanticipated, this usually results in a cancelled or partially performed examination that is unsatisfying for patients and institutions.

Because of new high-speed multidetector scanners, CT scanning has experienced a revival. The ability to gate these scans has allowed the production of elegant images previously not possible. At present, this requires sufficiently low heart rates (60–70 bpm) and the ability to breath-hold. CT offers the advantage of superior visualization in and around metallic implants, such as stents placed in the aorta for coarctation. CT also has the ability to visualize the coronaries and is beginning to approach the diagnostic sensitivity of angiography. This milestone is anticipated,

although it is yet to come to fruition. The large doses of radiation required to generate elegant images make serial CT examinations unattractive for the follow-up of young patients over the course of a lifetime.

### Cardiac catheterization

What is the role of catheterization? Is it only a dinosaur in the face of such advanced imaging? Is it barbaric to use catheters to measure pressures and inject dye directly into a cardiac chamber for fleeting seconds when a simple peripheral intravenous injection suffices for detailed cross-sectional imaging?

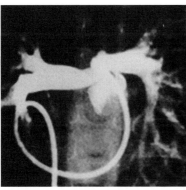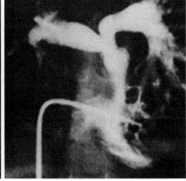

Fig. 21. Angiography for selective intervention on the branch pulmonary arteries can be most difficult because of overlapping of structures. No single projection is totally representative and multiple views frequently are required. In the left panel, a scout film is taken in the main pulmonary artery, and in the right, the right ventricle. Both images are taken in the cranial-LAO projection and in these examples clearly outline the outflow tracts and branch confluences. In the left panel, the dilated main pulmonary artery would have obscured the branch pulmonary artery confluence, and this cranial LAO (*left upper panel*) and caudal left LAT (*right upper panel*) nicely detail the anatomy for subsequent intervention.

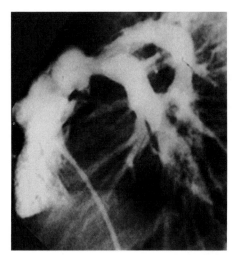

Fig. 22. The image is taken from a left-LAT projection with caudal tilt. This separates the proximal right and left pulmonary artery branches and details the main pulmonary artery. The outflow tract is foreshortened, and this view misleads operators when examining the diameter of the valve and the infundibulum. When examining the infundibulum and the diameter of the valve, a straight left LAT should be performed. In the caudal-LAT projection, the left pulmonary branch sweeps superiorly and toward the upper right corner of the image, whereas the left pulmonary artery appears more medial and in the center of the image. Using the left-LAT view, stents could be placed in each branch.

In counterpoint, catheterization is the only modality that provides the gold standard of pressure measurement in a vessel or chamber. In stark contrast to the complexities of the newest technology, the measurement of intracardiac pressures is simple, reliable, and reproducible. The assessment of the hemodynamic significance of a lesion never should be left to cross-sectional imaging and always verified by catheter. Some argue that an aortic valve never should be changed without a patient having had a catheter examination [11,12]. This may be interpreted as an old way of doing things by some, but by others it is a refreshing confirmation of the value of invasive imaging. Some send patients for operative correction of a defect without catheterization, but they may on occasion fall victim to this approach; an anomalous coronary may be missed and transected or ligated or an opportunity to address an unrecognized defect may be missed.

Catheterization is the only method to determine the pulmonary artery pressure and pulmonary vascular resistance accurately. These values are of utmost importance in many patients who have congenital heart disease. The time-honored practice of oximetry and shunt determination is a confirmatory piece of information and the weight placed on it is reflected in our current guidelines for intervention in congenital heart disease [13].

There are several situations where noninvasive imaging cannot provide the anatomic detail required for decision making. The recognition that noninvasive imaging may not assess the lumen of a pulmonary artery or collateral vessel after stenting reliably may lead to a further intervention that could improve patient quality of life.

Coronary angiography provides the only standard used to assess coronary lesions and their suitability for revascularization. The addition of invasive physiologic (coronary flow reserve) and imaging modalities (intravascular ultrasound) can make the resolution of a clinical question regarding lesion severity a straightforward issue. Diagnostic catheterization is alive and well in congenital heart disease.

## A look at today's interventions

Most adult congenital catheterization practices consist of approximately 70% intracardiac device implantation and approximately 30% other interventions. The world of device closure for ASDs is divided between ASD and PFO closure.

### Atrial septal defect closure

ASDs are present in approximately 0.317 of every 1000 live births [14]. A variety of devices has been used to close these defects, generally for the indication of right ventricular volume overload. The guidelines for these interventions are drawn from the Canadian and European grown up congenital heart recommendations [13,15]. ASD closure is a well-established and safe procedure. It can be performed on an outpatient basis with intracardiac echocardiography guidance and without the need for anesthesia or TEE. Such an approach presumes that patients have undergone a detailed TEE study to exclude associated abnormalities including, but not limited to, anomalous pulmonary venous return, additional secundum defects, fenestrations and sinus venosus defects, and the occasional septum primum defect. MRI and CT provide excellent detail with regard to pulmonary venous drainage but are somewhat lacking in specificity and sensitivity when it comes to small fenestrations or other small coexisting ASDs. A TEE also excludes left atrial thrombus and confirms the absence of significant valvular heart disease.

The most versatile device for this application is the Amplatzer Septal Occluder. It provides the benefit of a self-centering design (an issue with double umbrella devices) and is easy to implant. The residual leak rate after placement arguably is the lowest of any device and has the lowest rate of visible thrombus formation of any current device [16,17]. Many series of short- and medium-term results are published and demonstrate excellent results. Patients younger than age 40 generally have a complete return of their dilated right ventricular size to normal over the after 6 months (much of the improvement occurs immediately after the procedure) [18]. Many patients over 40 enjoy the same results. Most adults demonstrate objectively improved cardiopulmonary function after closure, including those who believe they were asymptomatic before the procedure [19–21]. There is a suggestion that patients who do not have arrhythmia before age 55 and who undergo closure may enjoy a lower risk of subsequently developing an arrhythmia [22].

Although a well-established procedure, the long-term safety of ASD device closure remains in question. Several late device erosions into the pericardium, aorta, or other structures are reported. The erosion rate is believed to involve approximately 0.1% of cases [23,24]. Caution is advised in cases of a deficient superior or aortic rim, with aggressive balloon sizing and device oversizing, and with aggressive maneuvers (push-pull) to verify device stability. Some advocate the abandonment of balloon sizing but have not presented data that this is a safer approach. The prospect of placing a large device (which results in remodeling and shrinkage of the right heart) into a small person remains a source of concern. Programs that do a lot of these procedures encounter a severe complication at some point.

### Patent foramen ovale closure

Although indications for ASD closure generally are accepted, the indications for closure of PFO for the secondary prevention of stroke are not. Although the evidence of benefit is limited, the number of procedures performed and the number of operators performing them continue to grow. Two major trials currently are under way examining whether or not device therapy is better or worse than medical therapy for secondary stroke prevention. These trials are slow to recruit patients and are in jeopardy of not being completed. The data arguing for closure rest mainly on evidence provided by single-center, retrospective, nonrandomized trials and with meta-analyses that have taken unfortunate liberties in interpretation and analysis [25,26]. The result is an unclear future for this procedure. Which patients will benefit from a percutaneous PFO closure procedure? Will it be only those who have atrial septal aneurysms or those who have multiple prior events? Will the complications of PFO closure, including arrhythmia, device thrombus formation, recurrent cerebrovascular events, or access complications, make this therapy less attractive than medical therapy? Will patients who have other risk factors for stroke, such as diabetes, or those who have nonsurgical carotid disease benefit from closure as a risk reduction strategy? The authors' policy regarding patients referred for PFO closure involves a detailed informed consent where many of these issues and questions are raised. The authors offer every appropriate patient entry into a randomized trial to help resolve these issues and tell each patient that there is no conclusive data to support closure at this time, a position supported by the American Academy of Neurology [27].

The treatment and follow-up of these patients who have ASD or PFO after device closure is another area of controversy. Most operators treat with ASA and clopidogrel for periods varying from 1 to 6 months or longer. The use of bubble studies to follow these patients who have transthoracic echocardiography (TTE) or TEE to "confirm closure" often is done without any evidence that this type of testing is important or helpful.

### Coarctation of the aorta

Stent placement for coarctation of the aorta is perhaps the most hazardous of all interventions performed in the catheter laboratory. Patients who have either native coarctation or previously treated coarctation may be candidates for treatment. In most patients, the intervention is indicated for a gradient of greater than 20 mm Hg across the coarctation site, usually in the setting of proximal hypertension. The authors also have intervened to treat pseudoaneurysms with covered stents and coils. Over the past several years, the authors have modified their approach to this procedure to improve its safety. They routinely obtain access from the right radial artery and the right femoral artery. This allows for simultaneous pressure measurement before and after stenting and immediate angiography after stent placement to rule out aortic dissection or perforation. This approach always has been one of direct stenting (primary stenting) in adults, without progressive balloon inflation until dissection is noted, and then stenting as advocated by others. The authors began with the use of the Palmaz Shatz P5014b stent (Jonhson & Johnson Interventional, Warren, New Jersey), which provided excellent radial strength but relatively poor flexibility, and then moved to the Genesis Biliary Stent (Johnson & Johnson), which provided less radial strength in return for flexibility. In follow-up, they have seen the Genesis stents buckle under the recoil of the aorta and also noted circumferential fractures. Most recently, they have used the CP PTFE-covered stent, which offers protection from aortic perforation and dissection, the most serious complications of this procedure. Also, for years they have been addressing the femoral access site as a source of complication by fully anticoagulating these patients and preclosing the access site using a suture-mediated closure device (Perclose AT Abbott Vascular Devices, Redwood City, California). The authors find that complete hemostasis is possible with few complications. The large arterial access (up to 14 Fr) required for this procedure remains a source of concern.

*Patent ductus arteriosus*

Patent ductus arteriosus (PDA) closure in adults usually is performed to reduce the risk of endarteritis. It is said that all ducts with an audible murmur should be closed. The intervention on PDAs has been facilitated greatly using the Amplatzer Duct Occluder (AGA Medical, Golden Valley, Minnesota). This is a well-designed device, which has little competition in the adult marketplace. This is a safe and quick procedure, which almost uniformly corrects the intended anatomic abnormality.

The authors, and others, have used this versatile device successfully to close perivalvular leaks around previously implanted mitral or aortic valve prostheses. They have limited these interventions to patients who have indications of severe mitral insufficiency associated with heart failure or transfusion-dependent hemolysis who are not surgical candidates or who are high-risk surgical candidates.

**A look at new and emerging interventions**

The next great series of innovations in cardiovascular intervention will be in valvular heart disease, such as the Bonhoeffer-Melody (Medtronic) stented pulmonary valve. In addition, percutaneous valve replacement has been achieved in humans with two different aortic valve prostheses. Pulmonary valve implantation initially will be offered to patients who have previously implanted conduits. At present, the largest percutaneous pulmonary valve is 22 mm. This size will limit its use to a select patient population for the time being. In short order, new stent designs or other interventional techniques should be expected to allow the treatment of patients who have larger conduits and native outflow tracts.

There likely will be a growth of hybrid surgical/interventional procedures that involve sophisticated imaging to examine physiology and anatomy immediately before and after repair. These hybrid procedures are performed rarely in the pediatric world and even more rarely in the adult setting. Until stented valves are able to treat the pulmonary insufficiency seen in aneurysmal outflow tracts in patients who have tetralogy, a novel hybrid approach can be envisioned. Surgeons may, through a minimally invasive approach, plicate the pulmonary artery or suture a percutaneous valve in place from the epicardial surface on a beating heart without cardiopulmonary bypass. Valves in the aortic position have been replaced via a periapical approach and a minithoracotomy, obviating femoral arteries large enough to handle a very large delivery system.

New structural heart disease suites, which take into account the need for operating room standard ventilation, anesthesia, and perfusion, will be required. There will continue to be a proliferation of minimally invasive procedures whereby surgery will facilitate the introduction of a device either percutaneously or directly on a beating heart, obviating cardiopulmonary bypass. Eventually, many of these procedures mostly will be percutaneous with surgeons and interventional colleagues working side by side in pursuit of the safest and most effective way to perform repair or replacement of a particular valve or vessel.

Surgical strategies for repair will take into account interventional advances, and childhood operations will be modified so that an interventional solution to a future reoperation may be possible. An example may be the performance of a modified hemi-Fontan to allow for catheter laboratory completion of the Fontan with a covered stent from the IVC to the PA. There may be implantation of fewer mechanical valves to permit the percutaneous implantation of tissue valves within failing surgically implanted stented tissue valves, which will serve as a matrix on which to build.

Guidance for these new procedures likely will involve 3-D imaging modalities and device manipulation and stabilization during the procedures, requiring that new expertise be developed. We live in interesting times, but they are certain to become more interesting, as structures as divinely inspired as the mitral valve become the substance of everyday catheter laboratory repair.

### The future role of diagnostic catheterization in the patients who have adult congenital heart disease

It is probable that what is known of diagnostic catheterization will change dramatically. A diagnostic catheterization may be expected to be performed in an imaging suite. Who the operator will be remains in question. A structural map may be created with cross-sectional imaging and then the navigation through tortuous pulmonary arteries or vessel occlusions or transeptally will be done with a 0.014 wire with a pressure transducer and a radiofrequency ablation assembly at its tip. The guidance of this small device may be solely magnetic. A nurse may place a peripheral intravenous line through which such a device is introduced. Oximetry may be measured in various chambers using similar wire tip technology without the need for blood sampling. The need for large devices, such as balloons and stents, will continue to require access to a large or central vein to permit their introduction.

Patients who have ACHD may no longer wait for different appointments for different imaging modalities. They will pass through a series of scanners in the course of an hour. The coronaries may be visualized via CT, the stenosed pulmonary artery and the gradient across it assessed by MR, followed by the crossing of the stenosis by a magnetically directed wire over which a balloon and stent will be introduced.

Will contrast angiography survive independent of interventional catheterization? It may not, at least not in its present form. Diagnostic catheterization will not disappear, but it will change. It will be less invasive, use less or no contrast, and may take place with the operator sitting in a control room using navigational equipment. To run an aircraft carrier, one need not turn a crank to drive the propeller.

### Summary

This short introduction to diagnostic and interventional heart catheterization in patients who have ACHD allows readers a point of departure for the invasive assessment and interventional treatment of the most common lesions. Many cases occur, however, that do not fall into a standard categorization and operators must be prepared to remember the basic principles outlined in this article and use creative approaches to define and treat the lesion optimally. Successful outcomes require patience, perseverance, and the learned experience of others.

### References

[1] Angelini P. Abnormalities of the coronary arteries. Normal and anomalous coronary arteries: definitions and classification. Am Heart J 1989;117: 418–34.

[2] Greenberg MA, Fish BG, Spindola-Franco H. Congenital anomalies of the coronary arteries. Radiol Clin North Am 1989;27:1127–46.

[3] Freedom RM, Culham JAG. Abnormalities of the coronary arteries. In: Freedom RM, Mawson JB, Yoo SJ, et al, editors. Congenital Heart Disease, textbook of angiocardiography. Armonk, NY: Futura Publishing Company, Inc.; 1997. p. 849–78.

[4] Ishikawa T, Brandt PWT. Anomalous origin of the left main coronary artery from the right anterior aortic sinus: angiographic definition of anomalous course. Am J Cardiol 1985;55(6):770–6.

[5] Serota H, Barth CW, Seuc CA, et al. Rapid identification of the course of anomalous coronary arteries in adults: the "dot and eye" method. Am J Cardiol 1990;65:891–8.

[6] Culham JAG. Physical principles of image formation and projections in angiocardiography. In: Freedom RM, Mawson JB, Yoo SJ, et al, editors. congenital heart disease textbook of angiocardiography. Armonk, NY: Futura Publishing; 1997. p. 39–93.

[7] Beekman RH 3rd, Hellenbrand WE, Lloyd TR, et al. ACCF/AHA/AAP recommendations for training in pediatric cardiology. Task force 3: training guidelines for pediatric cardiac catheterization and interventional cardiology endorsed by the Society for Cardiovascular Angiography and Interventions. J Am Coll Cardiol 2005;46:1388–90.

[8] Qureshi SA, Redington AN, Wren C, et al. Recommendations of the British Paediatric Cardiac Association for therapeutic cardiac catheterisation in

congenital cardiac disease. Cardiol Young 2000;10: 649–67.

[9] Ventricular septal defect. In: Freedom RM, Mawson JB, Yoo SJ, et al, editors. Congenital heart disease textbook of angiocardiography. Armonk, NY: Futura Publishing; 1997. p. 189–218.

[10] Brandt PW. Axially angled angiocardiography. Cardiovasc Intervent Radiol 1984;7:166–9.

[11] Griffith MJ, Carey C, Coltart DJ, et al. Inaccuracies of using aortic valve gradients alone to grade severity of aortic stenosis. Br Heart J 1989;62:372–8.

[12] Rahimtoola SH. Should patients with asymptomatic mild or moderate aortic stenosis undergoing coronary artery bypass surgery also have valve replacement for their aortic stenosis? Heart 2001;85:337–41.

[13] Therrien J, Dore A, Gersony W. CCS Consensus Conference 2001 update: recommendations for the Management of Adults with Congenital Heart Disease Part I. Can J Cardiol 2001;17:940–59.

[14] Ferencz C, Rubin JD, McCarter RJ, et al. Congenital heart disease: prevalence at livebirth. The Baltimore-Washington Infant Study. Am J Epidemiol 1985;121:31–6.

[15] Deanfield J, Thaulow E, Warnes C, et al. Management of grown up congenital heart disease. The Task force on the Management of Grown up Congenital Heart Disease of the European Society of Cardiology. Eur Heart J 2003;24:1035–84.

[16] Anzai H, Child J, Natterson B, et al. Incidence of thrombus formation on the CardioSEAL and the Amplatzer interatrial closure devices. Am J Cardiol 2004;93:426–31.

[17] Krumsdorf U, Ostermayer S, Billinger K, et al. Incidence and clinical course of thrombus formation on atrial septal defect and patient foramen ovale closure devices in 1,000 consecutive patients. J Am Coll Cardiol 2004;43:302–9.

[18] Veldtman GR, Razack V, Siu S, et al. Right ventricular form and function after percutaneous atrial septal defect device closure. J Am Coll Cardiol 2001;37:2108–13.

[19] Giardini A, Donti A, Formigari R, et al. Determinants of cardiopulmonary functional improvement after transcatheter atrial septal defect closure in asymptomatic adults. J Am Coll Cardiol 2004;43: 1886–91.

[20] Webb G, Horlick EM. Lessons from cardiopulmonary testing after device closure of secundum atrial septal defects: a tale of two ventricles. J Am Coll Cardiol 2004;43:1892–3.

[21] Brochu MC, Baril JF, Dore A, et al. Improvement in exercise capacity in asymptomatic and mildly symptomatic adults after atrial septal defect percutaneous closure. Circulation 2002;106:1821.

[22] Silversides CK, Siu SC, McLaughlin PR. Symptomatic atrial arrhythmias and transcatheter closure of atrial septal defects in adult patients. Heart 2004; 90:1194–8.

[23] Amin Z, Hijazi Z, Bass JL. Erosion of Amplatzer septal occluder device after closure of secundum atrial septal defects: review of registry of complications and recommendations to minimize future risk. Catheter Cardiovasc Interv 2004;63:496–502.

[24] Divekar A, Gaamangwe T, Shaikh N, et al. Cardiac perforation after device closure of atrial septal defects with the Amplatzer septal occluder. J Am Coll Cardiol 2005;45:1213–8.

[25] Windecker S, Wahl A, Nedeltchev K, et al. Comparison of medical treatment with percutaneous closure of patent foramen ovale in patients with cryptogenic stroke. J Am Coll Cardiol 2004;44:750–8.

[26] Landzberg MJ, Khairy P. Indications for the closure of patent foramen ovale. Heart 2004;90:219–24.

[27] Messe SR, Silverman IE, Kizer JR, et al. Practice parameter: recurrent stroke with patent foramen ovale and atrial septal aneurysm: report of the Quality Standards Subcommittee of the American Academy of Neurology. Neurology 2004;62:1042–50.

ELSEVIER
SAUNDERS

Cardiol Clin 24 (2006) 557–569

CARDIOLOGY
CLINICS

# The Geneticist's Role in Adult Congenital Heart Disease

Francois P. Bernier, MD*, Renee Spaetgens, MD

*Department of Medical Genetics, University of Calgary, Alberta Children's Hospital,
1820 Richmond Road, SW Calgary, AB T2T5C7, Canada*

The Human Genome Project promises to revolutionize our understanding and approach to human diseases. Specifically for congenital heart defects (CHDs), this project promises to identify the genes and pathways involved in normal cardiac development and to determine the impact of mutations in these genes in the pathogenesis of syndromic and nonsyndromic CHDs. For clinicians involved in the care of adults who have congenital heart disease, some of these advances in genetic knowledge are now being translated into clinical care, raising the question of what role this new era of genetic knowledge should have in the adult congenital heart disease (ACHD) clinic. The authors summarize the clinical and molecular advances relevant to the care and genetic counseling of ACHD patients and explore the role of genetic care providers in an ACHD clinic.

## The Role of genetics

Medical geneticists and genetic counselors are involved in the diagnosis, treatment, and counseling of patients who have or who are at risk for genetic diseases. In a pediatric setting, the focus is often on the short- and long-term medical and developmental outcomes for the affected child and on recurrence risks for the parents. In adult patients, the role expands to provide accurate information on the risk of having an affected child (recurrence risk) and what options, if any, are available for prenatal diagnosis. The accuracy of

this genetic counseling is primarily determined by the accuracy of the patient's diagnosis. For many patients in an ACHD clinic, their last medical genetics evaluation (if one was ever completed) may have taken place many years ago and before the significant advances that have occurred in the interim. For example, in many centers, newborns who have conotruncal CHDs are now routinely tested for 22q11 deletions, whereas few ACHD patients, if any, will likely have been tested. The importance of an accurate diagnosis is further exemplified by the fact that recurrence risks vary, in general, between zero (the risk associated, for example, with a teratogenic etiology) and 50% (the risk associated with an autosomal dominant condition). Providing inaccurate genetic counseling may not only falsely reassure or scare a prospective couple but also present a significant medical legal liability. In addition, the recurrence risk may apply not only to the risk of having a child with a CHD but also to a range of other birth defects or learning disabilities in those who have syndromic diagnoses. In an ACHD clinic, medical genetics can play a significant role in the clinical and genetic assessment of patients, with the goal of arriving at an accurate etiologic diagnosis to provide accurate counseling regarding recurrence risk and prenatal diagnosis and screening options.

## Toward an etiologic classification of congenital heart defects

Historically, CHDs were simply classified according to their physiologic effects. More recently, a developmentally oriented classification has been advocated by molecular biologists, particularly those interested in exploiting the power of model

* Corresponding author.

*E-mail address:* francois.bernier@calgaryhealthregion.ca
(F.P. Bernier).

systems for studying cardiac development given the apparent conservation of cardiac developmental steps in vertebrates [1]. Ultimately, an etiologic classification is anticipated. Historically, CHDs were classified as isolated or associated with a syndrome, with the former being mainly thought to be due to multifactorial inheritance with a minority resulting from single-gene, chromosomal, or teratogenic causes. Molecular advances are challenging this assumption, and it is anticipated that the large "multifactorial" group of patients may be much more etiologically heterogeneous [2]. Nevertheless, the assignment of an ACHD patient into one of the above etiologic categories remains an important clinical exercise.

### Genetics of isolated congenital heart disease

It has long been recognized that congenital heart disease tends to cluster in families. Most families demonstrate a multifactorial mode of inheritance, whereby the risk of congenital heart disease increases when one or more closely related family members is affected. A number of rare families who demonstrate a classic mendelian pattern of inheritance of isolated CHDs have recently helped in the identification of several single-gene causes of CHDs. Although their overall contribution to sporadic congenital heart disease is likely to be low, the hope is that their identification will provide knowledge about the underlying mechanisms of heart defects that could ultimately result in prevention or new therapeutics and improved clinical outcomes. To date, only a small number of single-gene causes of isolated heart defects have been identified, suggesting that CHDs in general are extremely heterogeneous and genetically complex.

Identification of single-gene causes of congenital heart disease has been largely accomplished with linkage studies in large families who have CHDs, from the study of recurrent chromosomal rearrangements, or based on the identification of the molecular etiology of rare genetic syndromes [3]. Described in the following paragraphs are a number of single-gene causes of isolated CHDs.

GATA4 encodes a transcription factor known to play a critical role in cardiogenesis. It is localized to chromosome 8p23.1. Pathogenic mutations were first identified in a large family who had isolated autosomal dominant ostium secundum atrial septal defects (ASDs) and have since been identified in other families who have isolated CHDs [4–7]. Although ASDs appear to be the most common type of heart defect associated with mutations in GATA4, additional defects have been seen, including ventricular septal defects (VSDs), atrioventricular septal defects (AVSDs), and pulmonary valve stenosis [4]. A novel mutation in GATA4 has also been found in two patients with isolated tetralogy of Fallot (TOF) [8]. The molecular mechanism by which GATA4 mutations cause septation defects (and others types of CHDs) remains to be elucidated, although it appears that at least some of the pathogenic mutations result in reduced transcriptional activation of downstream target genes [8]. The overall contribution of GATA4 mutations to familial CHD is probably modest. In one study, only 2 of 16 probands with familial ASD were found to have GATA4 mutations [5].

NKX2-5 encodes for a homeobox transcription factor that interacts functionally with GATA4. It is involved in the early determination of the heart field and may play a role in formation of the cardiac conduction system. Knockout animal models have demonstrated that the absence of NKX2-5 leads to acardia or severe defects in cardiac morphogenesis [9]. Mutations in NKX2-5 have been identified in several families who have familial nonsyndromic ASD with conduction defects [10]. It has also been less commonly associated with a variety of other heart defects including VSD, Ebstein's anomaly, TOF, fibromuscular subaortic stenosis, double-outlet right ventricle, and hypoplastic left heart. In addition, the NKX2-5 mutation can cause atrioventricular conduction block with or without associated congenital heart diseases, and all NKX2-5 mutation carriers are thought to have a lifelong risk for the development of heart block and sudden death. To date, approximately 20 heterozygous mutations in NKX2-5 have been reported to be associated with nonsyndromic congenital heart disease [11]. Most mutations result in protein truncation or an altered DNA binding domain. Overall, the impact of NKX2-5 mutations in sporadic isolated CHDs appears to be small [12].

Several other single-gene causes of congenital heart disease are known. Missense mutations in CRELD1, a cell adhesion molecule expressed during cardiac development, have been identified in patients who have nonsyndromic sporadic AVSDs [13]. Mutations in ZIC3, an X-linked transcription factor, have been found in sporadic and X-linked laterality defects, and less commonly in transposition of the great arteries (TGA) [14,15]. Mutations in JAG1, the gene that causes Alagille syndrome, have been identified in familial cases of isolated right-sided cardiac lesions [16]. Elastin mutations are seen in dominantly inherited isolated supraval-var aortic and pulmonic stenosis [17].

Molecular genetic testing for mutations in the abovementioned genes is not yet available on a clinical basis. As we learn more about the underlying genetic causes of congenital heart disease and as genetic testing becomes clinically available, important issues regarding genetic testing will become important. These issues include appropriate timing of testing, medical insurability, confidentiality, and cost of genetic testing. Clinical utility and relevance to patient management will need to be demonstrated before testing becomes routinely available.

## Teratogenic causes of congenital heart disease

Environmental factors also play an important role in the development of CHDs. A number of teratogens are known to be associated with CHDs, the most notable of which are maternal diabetes and alcohol. Heart defects that are the result of a teratogenic exposure are not associated with an increased risk of CHDs in siblings or offspring, assuming the exposure does not occur in subsequent pregnancies.

Fetuses born to mothers who have diabetes mellitus are at increased risk of heart defects as isolated malformations or in association with other features of diabetic embryopathy (ie, caudal regression). The risk of heart defects in mothers who have diabetes is 3% to 5% and is dependent on glycemic control. In those who have good glycemic control, the rates of CHDs are similar to the general population risk. The most common lesions associated with maternal diabetes are VSDs, coarctation of the aorta, and TGA. There is also an increased risk for laterality defects. The association of diabetes with heart defects suggests that this embryologic pathway is particularly susceptible to disruption by disturbances of glucose homeostasis. Other maternal medical conditions are also associated with risk for CHDs in offspring. Maternal rubella infection carries a 35% risk of heart defects, although widespread vaccination for rubella should prevent most congenital rubella infections and associated heart defects. Maternal systemic lupus erythematosis can cause complete heart block in a portion of the fetuses whose mothers carry specific autoantibodies (antiRo, antiLa). Maternal phenylketonuria is associated with approximately a 25% risk

of CHDs, particularly TOF. The risk of adverse outcome (including microcephaly and mental handicap) is related to the level of maternal serum phenylalanine. A phenylalanine-free diet and normal serum phenylalanine levels before conception and throughout pregnancy can reduce the risk of malformations to that of the general population.

Prenatal alcohol exposure increases the risk of CHD. VSD is the most common heart defect seen with alcohol exposure, but ASD, TOF, and a variety of other defects can occur. Major anomalies are more likely to occur with heavy alcohol consumption. Other common teratogens that can increase the risk of CHD include anticonvulsants, lithium, and retinoic acid. Prenatal retinoic acid exposure, for example, is associated with a 10% to 20% risk of conotruncal heart defects, in addition to multiple other malformations.

## Syndromic causes of congenital heart disease

Syndromic and chromosomal etiologies are an important cause of CHDs. About 3% to 5% of CHDs are associated with recognizable genetic syndromes [18], and a further significant portion are associated with other congenital malformations of unknown etiology. Although most syndrome diagnoses are made during infancy and childhood in a pediatric setting, review in a setting such as the ACHD clinic may lead to the diagnosis of an underlying genetic syndrome in adults who have subtle presentations or in adults not previously evaluated by a geneticist. CHDs are components of many genetic syndromes. Online Mendelian Inheritance in Man [19] lists over 300 syndromes including CHDs. Diagnosis of syndromic causes of congenital heart disease is important for a variety of reasons including appropriate management of and screening for other medical problems associated with a particular syndrome and for accurate counseling for recurrence risk for other family members and offspring of the affected individual. Common syndromic and chromosomal causes of congenital heart disease that might be encountered or diagnosed in an ACHD clinic are discussed in the following sections and summarized in Table 1.

### Aneuploidy syndromes

*Turner's syndrome*

Turner's syndrome, a chromosomal disorder affecting women, has considerable phenotypic

Table 1
Summary of common syndromes associated with cardiac anomalies

| Syndrome | Cardiac manifestations | Noncardiac manifestations | Etiology | Inheritance pattern |
|---|---|---|---|---|
| Turner's syndrome | (15%–50%) Predominantly left-sided lesions (ie, BAV, coarctation); risk for aortic root dilatation | Variable phenotype; short stature, gonadal dysgenesis, lymphedema, renal anomalies, normal intelligence but can have learning disability | Chromosomal (45, X karyotype and variants mosaicism, structurally abnormal X chromosome) | Sporadic; affected women are almost always infertile |
| Down syndrome | (50%) Perimembranous VSD, PDA, ASD, and AVSD are most common; 50% require surgical intervention | Dysmorphic facies, mental handicap; hearing and vision loss, early-onset dementia | Chromosomal trisomy for chromosome 21 (rarely Robertsonian translocation or mosaicism) | Usually sporadic; associated with late maternal age; infertility in affected adults |
| 22q11 microdeletion syndrome | (75%) Conotruncal malformations are most common; TOF in 20%; anomalies of major neck vessels are also common | Variable phenotype; palate defects, developmental delay/learning difficulties, dysmorphic facies, immune deficiency, hypocalcemia, psychiatric illness in adulthood | Microdeletion at 22q11.2 detectable with FISH (95%); ~90% de novo | Autosomal dominant; 50% risk to offspring |
| Williams syndrome | (80%–90%) SVAS in 75%; any artery may be narrowed; hypertension in adults | Dysmorphic facies, stellate iris, developmental delay, short stature, connective tissue abnormalities, hypercalcemia | Microdeletion at 7q11.12 involving the elastin gene detectable with FISH (99%); most are de novo | Autosomal dominant; 50% risk to offspring |
| Noonan's syndrome | (50%–90%) Pulmonic stenosis (20%–50%) Hypertrophic cardiomyopathy (20%–30%) | Variable phenotype, short stature, webbed neck, dysmorphic facies, varying developmental delay; cryptorchidism; coagulation defects | PTPN11 mutations in 50%; half of cases are de novo | Autosomal dominant; 50% risk to offspring |
| VATER association | (80%) CHD of any type and severity | Vertebral defects, anal atresia, TEF, renal and limb anomalies, normal intelligence | No specific recurring etiology | Sporadic; very small risk to offspring |

(*continued on next page*)

Table 1 (*continued*)

| Syndrome | Cardiac manifestations | Noncardiac manifestations | Etiology | Inheritance pattern |
|---|---|---|---|---|
| Holt-Oram syndrome | (75%) Ostium secundum ASD; VSD; conduction defects | Upper limb anomalies of varying degrees (especially radial ray) in 100% | *TBX5* mutation (70%); 15% familial | Autosomal dominant; 50% risk to offspring |
| Alagille syndrome | (80%–100%) Pulmonary valve, artery and branch PA most commonly affected; TOF in 7%–15% | Hepatic disease, dysmorphic facies, posterior embryotoxin, butterfly vertebrae, renal anomalies, neurovascular anomalies | *JAG1* mutation (70%) or deletion (~5%); 50%–70% of cases are de novo | Autosomal dominant; 50% risk to offspring |
| CHARGE syndrome | (60%–85%) Commonly right-sided and conotruncal lesions | Colobomas, growth failure, developmental delay, choanal atresia, genital hypoplasia, ear anomalies and hearing loss | *CHD7* mutation (60%) or deletion; most cases are de novo | Autosomal dominant; 50% risk to offspring but reduced fertility |

*Abbreviations:* BAV, bicuspid aortic valve; FISH, fluorescence in situ hybridization; PA, pulmonary artery; PDA, patent ductus arteriosus; SVAS, supravalvar aortic stenosis; TEF, tracheoesophageal fistula.

variation. Some patients may be diagnosed at birth with classic physical features of webbed neck, excess nuchal skin, and marked lymphedema. Other patients have only subtle features and may not be diagnosed until adolescence or adulthood when undergoing investigation for short stature, amenorrhea, or infertility. Common physical features of Turner's syndrome include short stature, gonadal dysgenesis, cardiovascular malformations, lymphedema (webbed neck, edema of the hands and feet), and structural renal abnormalities. Intelligence is normal but mild speech and language delays can occur and there tends to be a specific difficulty with spatial/perceptual skills. Gonadal dysgenesis results in delayed or absent secondary sexual characteristics and infertility in most women who have Turner's syndrome.

Cardiac anomalies are present in 15% to 50% of individuals who have Turner's syndrome. Left-sided lesions predominate, with bicuspid aortic valve being the most common defect. Coarctation of the aorta is seen in approximately 10% of cases. Hypoplastic left heart, VSD, anomalous pulmonary venous drainage, and conduction defects have also been seen [20]. Aortic root dilation is seen in 5% to 10% of women who have Turner's syndrome and can lead to aortic root dissection in adult life. Regular echocardiographic surveillance of aortic root diameter and appropriate screening/treatment of risk factors for dissection, such as hypertension, are important components of management of women who have Turner's syndrome during adulthood [21]. Close monitoring by a cardiologist during pregnancy (invariably achieved through assisted reproductive technology) is imperative because of the risk of rupture or dissection of the aorta in pregnancy [22].

Turner's syndrome is classically associated with a 45,X karyotype but can be seen with a variety of 45,X variants including 46,XX karyotypes with X chromosome structural abnormalities. Mosaicism (45,X/46,XX or 45,X/46,XY) is also frequently seen and seems to be associated with a milder phenotype. The prevalence of Turner's syndrome is 1 in 2500 live births, although prevalence in conceptuses is much higher because of the high rate of fetal death.

*Down syndrome*

Down syndrome is characterized by a variety of congenital malformations, characteristic facial features, minor physical differences, and mental handicap. It usually is easily diagnosed in the newborn period based on the presence of typical dysmorphic features that include brachycephaly, upslanting palpebral fissures, flat facial profile, single palmar crease, and sandal gap (wide space between the first and second toe). Cardiac anomalies are the most frequent type of birth defect in individuals who have Down syndrome, but various other congenital malformations are also seen. Duodenal atresia/stenosis and Hirschsprung's disease are the most common malformations after heart defects. Developmental delay is universal, and all affected individuals have some degree of mental handicap. Adults who have Down syndrome generally require supervised home and work environments. Median life expectancy is about 50 years. An important cause of this reduced life expectancy, apart from the contribution of increased mortality secondary to CHDs in infancy and childhood, is a very high rate of dementia with cognitive and neuropathologic findings identical to those seen in Alzheimer's disease.

Congenital heart disease is seen in about 50% of individuals who have Down syndrome. Half of those will have a serious CHD that requires surgical intervention. The most common heart defects are a perimembranous VSD, followed by patent ductus arteriosus and ASD. AVSD is the classic CHD seen in Down syndrome, occurring 100 times more frequently in Down syndrome than in the general population. Other types of complex heart disease are also seen. The presence, type, and severity of heart defects are important determinants of survival in individuals who have Down syndrome. Screening with echocardiography is part of the routine investigation of any infant/child who has a confirmed or a suspected diagnosis of Down syndrome.

Down syndrome is caused by the presence of an extra copy of chromosome 21, specifically region 21q22. Most cases of Down syndrome are the result of standard trisomy 21. Five percent of cases are due to Robertsonian translocations involving chromosome 21 (which may or may not be familial) or to trisomy 21 mosaicism. Increased maternal age is the single most important risk factor for trisomy 21. Men who have Down syndrome are infertile. Despite normal sexual development in girls, there are only a small number of cases of documented fertility in women. Risk of recurrence in offspring is therefore generally immaterial, although it would be increased over that of the general population.

## Microdeletion syndromes

### 22q11 microdeletion syndrome

The 22q11 microdeletion syndrome is the most commonly occurring microdeletion syndrome in humans [23]. It goes by many names (partly dependent on which features are present in an individual): velocardiofacial syndrome, Shprintzen's syndrome, DiGeorge syndrome or sequence, and conotruncal anomaly face syndrome. This condition has a highly variable range of expression. Over 180 different clinical features have been reported in individuals who have 22q11 microdeletion. Affected individuals may have many features of the syndrome or only one or two features with subtle facial dysmorphism, making diagnosis difficult. The frequency in the general population is thought to about 1 in 4000, but this figure likely represents an underestimate given the under-recognition of mild cases. The most common findings in the 22q11 microdeletion syndrome are CHDs; palate abnormalities including velopharyngeal insufficiency, submucosal cleft palate, and frank cleft palate; characteristic facial features; and learning difficulties or developmental delay [24]. Other manifestations are immune deficiency (thymic hypoplasia), hypocalcemia (parathyroid hypoplasia), feeding difficulties, renal anomalies, and hearing loss. Individuals who have the 22q11 deletion are at increased risk for psychiatric illness in adulthood. Typical facial features are subtle but appear in most affected individuals. These features include a long face and tubular shaped nose. Micrognathia, mild hypertelorism, and hooded eyelids may also be seen.

CHDs occur in about 75% of individuals who have 22q11 microdeletion syndrome. The conotruncal malformations are the most common types of heart defects. TOF occurs in approximately 20% of individuals. Other conotruncal lesions include interrupted aortic arch, VSD, and truncus arteriosus [23]. In many centers, infants who have TOF, interrupted aortic arch, and truncus arteriosus are routinely screened for the 22q11 microdeletion. Nonconotruncal lesions can also occur in this condition. Bicuspid aortic valve, ASD, TGA, and anomalous origin of the coronary artery have been reported. Anomalies of the internal carotid arteries and other major neck vessels are also a common finding.

The 22q11 microdeletion results from a deletion of about 3 megabases (Mb) on the distal end of the long arm of chromosome 22. A small proportion of affected individuals have smaller 1.5-Mb deletions. A deletion is visible on a routine high-resolution karyotype in about 15% of cases. The rest of the cases are diagnosable only with fluorescence in situ hybridization (FISH) using a probe specific for this region. FISH studies detect deletions in over 95% of affected individuals. The deletion results in haploinsuffiency for over 30 genes in a typical 3-Mb deletion. Of these genes, TBX1 is believed to be responsible for most heart and vascular anomalies [25,26]. Ninety-three percent of individuals who have the 22q11 microdeletion have de novo deletions. The risk of 22q11 deletions in offspring of affected individuals is 50%. The severity of the condition in offspring or siblings is variable and cannot be predicted based on the phenotype of the proband. It is not uncommon to diagnose a mildly affected parent after the birth of a more severely affected infant.

*Williams syndrome*

Williams syndrome is characterized by dysmorphic facial features, developmental delay, short stature, and CHDs. A range of connective tissue abnormalities including hoarse voice, inguinal/umbilical hernia, bowel/bladder diverticulae, rectal prolapse, joint limitation or laxity, and soft, lax skin are frequently observed. Hypercalcemia or hypercalciuria are common. The range of intellectual impairment is wide, ranging from low average intelligence to severe mental retardation. The cognitive profile is unique, with particular strengths in verbal language and memory skills in contrast to very poor visuospatial abilities. The behavioral phenotype is characterized by anxiety, attention problems, and overfriendliness to strangers. The term "cocktail party" personality is frequently used to describe these patients. Distinctive facial characteristics include bitemporal narrowing, periorbital fullness, short nose, full nasal tip, midface hypoplasia, long philtrum, full lips, wide mouth, and prominent earlobes. Adults typically have a long face and neck resulting in a more gaunt appearance. Also present is a stellate/lacy iris pattern.

The cardiovascular features of this condition are secondary to elastin arteriopathy. Cardiac abnormalities are seen in 80% to 90% of individuals. Supravalvar aortic stenosis (SVAS) is the most clinically significant and most common cardiovascular finding, occurring in about 75% of affected individuals. SVAS can take the form of a discrete narrowing above the valve (hourglass stenosis) or a more diffuse long-segment aortic hypoplasia. These lesions tend to be progressive. Thirty percent to 40% of individuals who have SVAS eventually require surgical correction. Although the aorta is most frequently involved, any artery may be narrowed. Supravalvar pulmonic stenosis, peripheral pulmonic stenosis, renal artery stenosis, and coronary artery involvement can be seen. Unlike the aortic lesions, however, the pulmonary lesions tend to regress with time. Hypertension is common in adolescents and adults. Mitral valve prolapse and aortic insufficiency have also been reported in adults. In general, cardiovascular disease tends to be more severe in men.

Williams syndrome is caused by a submicroscopic deletion of 7q11.23. The commonly deleted region spans 1.5 Mb, and 21 genes have so far been mapped within this region. Many of the manifestations (arteriopathy, hoarse voice, hernias, and connective tissue abnormalities) of Williams syndrome are due to deletion (and therefore haploinsufficiency) of the elastin gene. FISH studies demonstrate deletion of the elastin gene in 99% of individuals who have Williams syndrome. Families who have isolated familial SVAS typically have point mutations within the elastin gene and do not demonstrate deletions with FISH. Most cases of Williams syndrome are de novo. An affected individual has a 50% chance of passing the condition to his/her offspring. The prevalence of Williams syndrome is about 1 in 10,000 live births.

**Single-gene disorders**

*Noonan syndrome*

Noonan syndrome is a relatively common syndrome characterized by short stature, CHDs, broad or webbed neck, pectus deformities, varying degrees of developmental delay, cryptorchidism in male patients, and dysmorphic facial features. Facial appearance changes over time and is most subtle in the adult. Key features irrespective of age include low-set posteriorly rotated ears with fleshy helices, vivid blue or blue-green irides, widely spaced eyes with epicanthal folds, and thick or droopy eyelids. Other features of this syndrome include a variety of ocular abnormalities, renal anomalies (generally mild), and scoliosis. Various coagulation defects may occur in Noonan syndrome and affect approximately one third of individuals. The coagulopathy may range from severe surgical hemorrhage to clinically mild bruising or to laboratory anomalies with no clinical sequelae. Routine screening for coagulopathy at the time of diagnosis should include prothrombin time, partial thromboplastin time, and platelet count. Acetylsalicylic acid should be avoided in those who have laboratory or clinical evidence of coagulopathy, and physicians should be aware of the potential for prolonged bleeding in those undergoing surgical procedures. Men who have Noonan syndrome are frequently infertile secondary to cryptorchidism. The prevalence of Noonan syndrome is about 1 in 2500, and mild cases are often unrecognized.

The frequency of congenital heart disease in individuals who have Noonan syndrome is 50% to 90%. The frequency of Noonan syndrome among children who have congenital heart disease is approximately 1.4%. A stenotic, often dysplastic, pulmonary valve is the most common heart defect in Noonan syndrome and is seen in 20% to 50% of individuals. Seven percent of those who have valvular pulmonary stenosis have an underlying diagnosis of Noonan syndrome. Dysplastic valves, with reduced mobility rather than fusion of valve commissures, are rare in non-Noonan individuals. Hypertrophic cardiomyopathy is also a relatively frequent cardiovascular finding in Noonan syndrome, occurring in about 20% to 30% of affected individuals [27]. It can range from mild localized ventricular septal hypertrophy to severe hypertrophic cardiomyopathy associated with significant mortality. The cardiomyopathy can present in utero, during infancy, or during childhood. Clinical and echocardiographic features are identical to nonsyndromic hypertrophic cardiomyopathy, although it appears that arrhythmia and sudden death are less common in the hypertrophic cardiomyopathy associated with Noonan syndrome. Other cardiac defects frequently seen in this condition include ASD, VSD, supravalvar pulmonic stenosis, branch pulmonary artery stenosis, TOF, coarctation of the aorta, and even partial AVSDs.

Noonan syndrome is an autosomal dominant condition demonstrating marked variability of expression. About half of the cases arise de novo. Half of the cases are familial, and it is not uncommon to diagnose Noonan syndrome in a mildly affected parent following the diagnosis of an affected infant or child. Missense mutations in the *PTPN11* gene have been identified in about 50% of individuals who have Noonan syndrome [28]. Sequence analysis of *PTPN11* is available on a clinical basis.

*Holt-Oram syndrome*

Holt-Oram syndrome is the best recognized of the heart-hand syndromes. It is characterized by cardiac defects and upper-limb anomalies of variable severity. Skeletal defects involve the upper limbs exclusively and are usually bilateral and asymmetric. They typically involve the radial ray. Defects range from mild involvement with clinodactyly (curved fingers), limited supination, or narrow sloping shoulders to more severe defects with absent, hypoplastic, or triphalangeal thumb. At the most severe end of the spectrum are reduction deformities that may include any part of the upper limb. The left side is typically more severely affected than the right side. At a minimum, all affected individuals have an abnormal carpal bone that may be the only evidence of disease. Posterior hand radiographs can identify such defects. The broad range of severity of these findings is such that some individuals who have the mildest upper-limb malformations and no or only mild CHDs may escape diagnosis. In general, the manifestations of Holt-Oram syndrome tend to be more severe in women.

The CHDs most commonly observed in Holt-Oram syndrome are ostium secundum ASD and VSD, especially those occurring in the muscular trabeculated septum. More severe cardiac defects such as hypoplastic left heart and total anomalous pulmonary veins have been reported. CHDs are seen in about 75% of affected individuals, and a further proportion of affected individuals may have nonspecific ECG abnormalities. Individuals who have Holt-Oram syndrome, with or without a congenital heart malformation, are at risk for cardiac conduction defects including complete heart block and atrial fibrillation. There appears to be some correlation between the severity of the upper-limb defect and the severity of the cardiac lesion.

Holt-Oram syndrome is an autosomal dominant disorder caused by heterozygous mutations in the transcription factor TBX5 [29,30]. Over 70% of individuals who meet strict diagnostic criteria (ie, upper-limb defect plus personal or family history of structural or conductive heart disease) have a *TBX5* mutation [31]. Clinical testing is available for *TBX5* mutations. The estimated frequency of Holt-Oram syndrome is 1 in 100,000 births. About 85% of cases are the result of new mutations. There is significant variable expressivity observed in individuals who have Holt-Oram syndrome, within and among families who have the same mutation. The phenotype of affected offspring, therefore, cannot be accurately predicted. In general, of those who have inherited a *TBX5* mutation, one third have a severe reduction defect of the upper limb (ie, absent thumb), and 5% have phocomelia.

*Alagille syndrome*

Alagille syndrome is a highly variable, multisystem condition involving the liver, heart, eyes, face, and skeleton. Bile duct paucity has traditionally been required for diagnosis, and hepatic presentation with conjugated hyperbilirubinemia or cholestasis, often in the neonatal period, is typical. Progression to cirrhosis or liver failure necessitating transplant occurs in about 20% of affected individuals. The classic eye finding is posterior embryotoxin, an eye abnormality that results in a white ring at the periphery of the cornea and is a benign anterior chamber finding. Butterfly vertebrae (clefting of the vertebral body) are seen in about 50% of individuals but are rarely symptomatic. Less frequently encountered problems include pancreatic insufficiency and a variety of structural renal abnormalities. Neurovascular anomalies predisposing to intracranial bleeds are seen in about 15% of individuals. The overall mortality rate is about 10% and attributable to cardiac and liver disease and vascular accidents. Characteristic facial features are seen in most individuals, although they tend to be more subtle in adulthood. Features include prominent forehead, pointed chin, deep-set eyes, hypertelorism, and bulbous nose.

Cardiac involvement occurs in 80% to 100% of individuals who have Alagille syndrome. Most heart defects are hemodynamically insignificant. The pulmonary vasculature (including valve, artery, and branches) is most frequently involved. The most common defect is peripheral pulmonary stenosis, which tends not to be progressive. Other heart defects include TOF, VSD, ASD, aortic stenosis, and aortic coarctation. The clinical outcomes of those who have TOF and Alagille syndrome may be poor compared with those who have typical isolated TOF [32]. TOF occurs in 7% to 16% of individuals who have Alagille syndrome.

Alagille syndrome is an autosomal dominant condition. It is caused by mutations in the *JAG1* gene [30,33]. JAG1 is a cell surface protein that functions in the notch signaling pathway. Mutations in *JAG1* are identified in about 70% of clinically affected individuals [34]. Deletions of the *JAG1* gene, identifiable with FISH studies, are found in a further 5% to 7% of individuals who have Alagille syndrome. Larger deletions are associated with a more severe phenotype and additional clinical features such as developmental delay or hearing loss. Clinical testing by sequence analysis for point mutations and FISH analysis for deletions is available. Fifty percent to 70% of *JAG1* mutations are de novo. The molecular characterization of Alagille syndrome has shown that affected individuals may have only very subtle or isolated findings. Such patients are often diagnosed only following the diagnosis of a more classically affected offspring. Risk to offspring of an affected parent is 50%. No genotype/phenotype correlations have been found, so the severity of clinical features cannot be predicted based on genotype or the degree to which a parent is affected. The prevalence of Alagille syndrome is 1 in 70,000 to 1 in 100,000, although this range may be an underestimate.

*CHARGE syndrome*

CHARGE syndrome is a multiple congenital anomaly syndrome characterized by colobomas of the iris, retina, or optic disc; CHD; postnatal growth failure; developmental delay; choanal atresia; genital hypoplasia (particularly in men); and ear abnormalities that can include external and internal ear anomalies and hearing loss. Other relatively common features are facial palsy, renal anomalies, orofacial clefts, and tracheoesophageal fistula.

CHDs are seen in about 60% to 85% of individuals who have CHARGE syndrome. The severity and the spectrum of heart defects vary, although there appears to be a preponderance of right-sided lesions and conotruncal defects. About 75% of heart defects in patients who have CHARGE syndrome require surgical intervention.

CHARGE syndrome was recently discovered to be caused by mutations in the *CHD7* gene, which codes for a chromodomain helicase DNA binding protein [35]. Mutations in *CHD7* are found in about 60% of patients meeting diagnostic criteria for CHARGE syndrome. Whole gene deletions of *CHD7* are also reported. Clinical testing by sequence analysis for point mutations and FISH analysis for deletions are available. Most mutations and deletions are de novo. Many patients who have CHARGE syndrome, particularly men, have delayed or absent puberty and infertility. Of those who reproduce, the risk to offspring is 50%. The prevalence of CHARGE syndrome is estimated to be about 1 in 9000 to 1 in 12,000.

### Associations

*VATER association*

VATER association is a sporadic constellation of congenital malformations that occur together more often than expected by chance alone. It is a diagnosis of exclusion. VATER is characterized by a combination of vertebral defects, anal atresia, CHDs, tracheoesophageal fistula, renal anomalies, and limb defects. Rarely do individuals have all of the above anomalies. Development and intelligence are normal. Dysmorphic facies are not present. The prognosis of the condition depends on which features are present, their severity, and the degree to which they can be treated.

CHDs are the most common finding in the VATER association. Approximately 80% of affected individuals have cardiac involvement. Heart defects can be of any type and severity.

No specific recurring etiology has been established for VATER. The prevalence is 1.6 in 10,000. There does not appear to be a large risk for recurrence in siblings or offspring of individuals who have VATER association.

### Genetics and adult patients who have congenital heart disease

In addition to providing cardiac care, ACHD clinics can play an important role in identifying patients who might benefit from additional genetic assessment and counseling. This counseling may be particularly relevant for patients of reproductive age. Determining whether patients are interested in obtaining information on recurrence risks should be explored with all ACHD patients [36].

Additional patients who might benefit from further assessment include those who have non–CHD-related medical problems, congenital anomalies, or learning/cognitive deficits. It may be more difficult for some clinicians to consider whether the patient has a more subtle pattern of physical features that might suggest the presence of an

underlying syndrome. For example, the hypertelorism (wide spacing of the eyes) seen in Noonan syndrome can vary from subtle to striking. Screening for patients who have a family history of CHDs should also be undertaken by asking whether any first-degree (parents, siblings, and children) or second-degree (grandparents, aunts/uncles, and nieces/nephews) relatives have a history of CHDs [2]. The presence of a single affected third-degree relative (eg, first cousin) is unlikely to be significant. A family history of major malformations, unexplained infant deaths, or significant learning/cognitive disabilities could be an indication that an underlying syndrome is segregating in the family (Box 1).

The role of 22q11 testing merits specific attention. Beauchesne and colleagues [37] identified six patients who had 22q11 deletions in a cohort of 103 consecutive adults who had high-risk CHD lesions (prevalence, 5.8%). In particular, they noted that patients often had few if any features that might have otherwise identified them as being at higher risk for 22q11 deletions. They advocated 22q11 testing in all patients who have high-risk lesions, which is a view supported by other investigators [2,37]. Patients who have 22q11 deletions should be screened for associated

---

**Box 1. Checklist for identifying adult congenital heart disease patients who might benefit from genetic assessment and counseling**

☐ Potential parents
☐ Unexplained medical conditions (eg, short stature, cholestasis, immune deficiency, psychiatric illness, hearing loss)
☐ Noncardiac malformations
☐ Facial dysmorphism
☐ Learning or cognitive disabilities
☐ 22q11 deletion status unknown in a patient who has a high-risk CHD (eg, outflow tract anomaly, pulmonary atresia/stenosis, tricuspic atresia, transposition)
☐ Family history of
  ☐ CHDs
  ☐ Major malformations
  ☐ Unexplained infant deaths or
  ☐ Significant learning/cognitive disabilities

medical problems in a genetics clinic or a multidisciplinary 22q11deletion clinic (if one is available locally) and offered further genetic counseling.

## Recurrence risks

Patients identified as being of reproductive age but for whom the remaining screening questions are normal likely have isolated CHDs and should be counseled regarding their specific recurrence risk, recognizing that limited and at-times conflicting data are available on recurrence risks (Table 2) [38,39]. Recurrence risks for offspring are higher than sibling recurrence risks, and for many CHDs, women appear to have a higher recurrence risk than men. The reason for the latter finding remains unknown. For most patients who have an isolated nonfamilial CHD, quoting a recurrence risk of 5% to 6% for women and 2% to 3% for men is appropriate until further data on CHD-specific recurrence risks become available. The recurrence risk for syndromic patients who have autosomal dominant conditions is 50%; for recessive conditions, the risk will depend on the carrier frequency in the population but will usually be quite low (see Table 1).

## Prenatal testing and screening

Women at increased risk of having a child who has a CHD are offered fetal echocardiography at 18 to 20 weeks' gestation [40]. Fetal nuchal translucency measurement between 11 and 14 weeks' gestation is a good screening test for CHD because the prevalence of CHD increases exponentially with fetal nuchal translucency thickness [41]. For patients at particularly high risk, early fetal echocardiography (11–13 weeks) can be considered if the expertise is available. Invasive prenatal, molecular, or cytogenetic testing following amniocentesis or chorionic villus sampling is available to patients who have identified single-gene or cytogenetic etiologies for their CHD. The offering of these later investigations should be accompanied by genetic counseling.

## Models of genetic service in adult congenital heart disease clinics

No literature could be identified by the authors on the subject of models of genetic service provision to patients who have ACHD. Most ACHD clinics refer to local genetic clinics, but some clinics have developed multidisciplinary care models. This latter model would likely promote more integrated care. In a recent survey of cardiologists and clinical geneticists regarding the provision of genetic services to hypertrophic cardiomyopathy patients, the majority of both groups indicated they preferred a model in which each group was responsible for specific steps of a cardiogenetic assessment [42]. With respect to ACHD patients, cardiologists may well be willing to undertake screening of appropriate patients to refer to genetics while leaving the further assessment and counseling of identified patients to genetics. ACHD clinics should nevertheless consider the inclusion of genetic care providers in the development of local care pathways and work toward multidisciplinary models of care.

Table 2
Risk of recurrence in offspring of parents who have congenital heart defects

| CHD | Risk to offspring (%) | | | |
| | 1994 Meta-analysis [38] | | 1998 British collaborative study [39] | |
| | Of women | Of men | Of women | Of men |
| --- | --- | --- | --- | --- |
| Atrioventicular septal defect | 11.6 | 4.3 | 7.9 | 7.7 |
| Aortic stenosis | 8.0 | 3.8 | | |
| Coarctation of the aorta | 6.3 | 3.0 | | |
| Pulmonary stenosis | 5.3 | 3.5 | | |
| Atrial septal defect | 6.1 | 3.5 | | |
| Ventricular septal defect | 6.0 | 3.6 | | |
| Persistent ductus arteriosus | 4.1 | 2.0 | | |
| Tetralogy of Fallot | 2.0 | 1.4 | 4.5 | 1.6 |
| Transposition great arteries | | | | |
| Anomalous pulmonary venous drainage | | | 5.9 | |
| Abnormal situs and other abnormal connections | | | 7.1 | 15.4 |
| All CHDs | 5.8 | 3.1 | 5.7 | 2.2 |

## Summary

With improved treatment of CHDs, patients now frequently survive to adulthood. CHDs are etiologically heterogeneous; however, there is significant evidence that genes play an important role in the etiology of most CHDs. Most ACHD patients have a recurrence risk of between 2% and 50%. Although the realization that they face a recurrence risk may not alter the reproductive plans of many patients, some may appreciate frank discussions regarding their risks and their reproductive options. Medical geneticists can play in important role in the identification, assessment, and counseling of at-risk ACHD patients and should be included as part of the multidisciplinary team caring for this patient population.

## References

[1] Pelech AN, Broeckel U. Toward the etiologies of congenital heart diseases. Clin Perinatol 2005; 32(4):825–44 [vii].

[2] Goldmuntz E. The genetic contribution to congenital heart disease. Pediatr Clin North Am 2004;51(6): 1721–37 [x].

[3] Grossfeld PD. The genetics of congenital heart disease. J Nucl Cardiol 2003;10(1):71–6.

[4] Garg V, Kathiriya IS, Barnes R, et al. GATA4 mutations cause human congenital heart defects and reveal an interaction with TBX5. Nature 2003; 424(6947):443–7.

[5] Hirayama-Yamada K, Kamisago M, Akimoto K, et al. Phenotypes with GATA4 or NKX2.5 mutations in familial atrial septal defect. Am J Med Genet A 2005;135(1):47–52.

[6] Okubo A, Miyoshi O, Baba K, et al. A novel GATA4 mutation completely segregated with atrial septal defect in a large Japanese family. J Med Genet 2004;41(7):e97.

[7] Sarkozy A, Conti E, Neri C, et al. Spectrum of atrial septal defects associated with mutations of NKX2.5 and GATA4 transcription factors. J Med Genet 2005;42(2):e16.

[8] Nemer G, Fadlalah F, Usta J, et al. A novel mutation in the GATA4 gene in patients with tetralogy of Fallot. Hum Mutat 2006;27(3):293–4.

[9] Ueyama T, Kasahara H, Ishiwata T, et al. Myocardin expression is regulated by Nkx2.5, and its function is required for cardiomyogenesis. Mol Cell Biol 2003;23(24):9222–32.

[10] Schott JJ, Benson DW, Basson CT, et al. Congenital heart disease caused by mutations in the transcription factor NKX2–5. Science 1998;281(5373):108–11.

[11] McElhinney DB, Geiger E, Blinder J, et al. NKX2.5 mutations in patients with congenital heart disease. J Am Coll Cardiol 2003;42(9):1650–5.

[12] Hobbs CA, Cleves MA, Keith C, et al. NKX2.5 and congenital heart defects: a population-based study. Am J Med Genet A 2005;134(2):223–5.

[13] Robinson SW, Morris CD, Goldmuntz E, et al. Missense mutations in CRELD1 are associated with cardiac atrioventricular septal defects. Am J Hum Genet 2003;72(4):1047–52.

[14] Gebbia M, Ferrero GB, Pilia G, et al. X-linked situs abnormalities result from mutations in ZIC3. Nat Genet 1997;17(3):305–8.

[15] Ware SM, Peng J, Zhu L, et al. Identification and functional analysis of ZIC3 mutations in heterotaxy and related congenital heart defects. Am J Hum Genet 2004;74(1):93–105.

[16] Krantz ID, Smith R, Colliton RP, et al. Jagged1 mutations in patients ascertained with isolated congenital heart defects. Am J Med Genet 1999;84(1): 56–60.

[17] Tassabehji M, Metcalfe K, Donnai D, et al. Elastin: genomic structure and point mutations in patients with supravalvular aortic stenosis. Hum Mol Genet 1997;6(7):1029–36.

[18] Meberg A, Otterstad JE, Froland G, et al. Outcome of congenital heart defects–a population-based study. Acta Paediatr 2000;89(11):1344–51.

[19] Online Mendelian Inheritance in Man. OMIM. McKusick-Nathans Institute for Genetic Medicine, Johns Hopkins University (Baltimore, MD) and National Center for Biotechnology Information, National Library of Medicine (Bethesda, MD), 2000. Available at: http://www.ncbi.nlm.nih.gov/omim/. Accessed March 15, 2006.

[20] Mazzanti L, Cacciari E. Congenital heart disease in patients with Turner's syndrome. Italian Study Group for Turner Syndrome (ISGTS). J Pediatr 1998;133(5):688–92.

[21] Elsheikh M, Casadei B, Conway GS, et al. Hypertension is a major risk factor for aortic root dilatation in women with Turner's syndrome. Clin Endocrinol (Oxf) 2001;54(1):69–73.

[22] Karnis MF, Zimon AE, Lalwani SI, et al. Risk of death in pregnancy achieved through oocyte donation in patients with Turner syndrome: a national survey. Fertil Steril 2003;80(3):498–501.

[23] Perez E, Sullivan KE. Chromosome 22q11.2 deletion syndrome (DiGeorge and velocardiofacial syndromes). Curr Opin Pediatr 2002;14(6): 678–83.

[24] Antshel KM, Kates WR, Roizen N, et al. 22q11.2 deletion syndrome: genetics, neuroanatomy and cognitive/behavioral features keywords. Child Neuropsychol 2005;11(1):5–19.

[25] Merscher S, Funke B, Epstein JA, et al. TBX1 is responsible for cardiovascular defects in velo-cardio-facial/DiGeorge syndrome. Cell 2001;104(4): 619–29.

[26] Yagi H, Furutani Y, Hamada H, et al. Role of TBX1 in human del22q11.2 syndrome. Lancet 2003; 362(9393):1366–73.

[27] Nishikawa T, Ishiyama S, Shimojo T, et al. Hypertrophic cardiomyopathy in Noonan syndrome. Acta Paediatr Jpn 1996;38(1):91–8.

[28] Tartaglia M, Mehler EL, Goldberg R, et al. Mutations in PTPN11, encoding the protein tyrosine phosphatase SHP-2, cause Noonan syndrome. Nat Genet 2001;29(4):465–8.

[29] Basson CT, Bachinsky DR, Lin RC, et al. Mutations in human TBX5 [corrected] cause limb and cardiac malformation in Holt-Oram syndrome. Nat Genet 1997;15(1):30–5.

[30] Li L, Krantz ID, Deng Y, et al. Alagille syndrome is caused by mutations in human Jagged1, which encodes a ligand for Notch1. Nat Genet 1997;16(3):243–51.

[31] McDermott DA, Bressan MC, He J, et al. TBX5 genetic testing validates strict clinical criteria for Holt-Oram syndrome. Pediatr Res 2005;58(5):981–6.

[32] McElhinney DB, Krantz ID, Bason L, et al. Analysis of cardiovascular phenotype and genotype-phenotype correlation in individuals with a JAG1 mutation and/or Alagille syndrome. Circulation 2002;106(20):2567–74.

[33] Oda T, Elkahloun AG, Pike BL, et al. Mutations in the human Jagged1 gene are responsible for Alagille syndrome. Nat Genet 1997;16(3):235–42.

[34] Krantz ID, Colliton RP, Genin A, et al. Spectrum and frequency of jagged1 (JAG1) mutations in Alagille syndrome patients and their families. Am J Hum Genet 1998;62(6):1361–9.

[35] Vissers LE, van Ravenswaaij CM, Admiraal R, et al. Mutations in a new member of the chromodomain gene family cause CHARGE syndrome. Nat Genet 2004;36(9):955–7.

[36] Uebing A, Steer PJ, Yentis SM, et al. Pregnancy and congenital heart disease. BMJ 2006;332(7538):401–6.

[37] Beauchesne LM, Warnes CA, Connolly HM, et al. Prevalence and clinical manifestations of 22q11.2 microdeletion in adults with selected conotruncal anomalies. J Am Coll Cardiol 2005;45(4):595–8.

[38] Nora JJ. From generational studies to a multilevel genetic-environmental interaction. J Am Coll Cardiol 1994;23(6):1468–71.

[39] Burn J, Brennan P, Little J, et al. Recurrence risks in offspring of adults with major heart defects: results from first cohort of British collaborative study. Lancet 1998;351(9099):311–6.

[40] Cohen MS, Frommelt MA. Does fetal diagnosis make a difference? Clin Perinatol 2005;32(4):877–90 [viii].

[41] Atzei A, Gajewska K, Huggon IC, et al. Relationship between nuchal translucency thickness and prevalence of major cardiac defects in fetuses with normal karyotype. Ultrasound Obstet Gynecol 2005;26(2):154–7.

[42] van Langen IM, Birnie E, Schuurman E, et al. Preferences of cardiologists and clinical geneticists for the future organization of genetic care in hypertrophic cardiomyopathy: a survey. Clin Genet 2005;68(4):360–8.

ELSEVIER
SAUNDERS

Cardiol Clin 24 (2006) 571–585

CARDIOLOGY
CLINICS

# The Anesthesiologist's Role in Adults with Congenital Heart Disease

Jane Heggie, MD, FRCP, Jacek Karski, MD, FRCP*

*Department of Anesthesia, Toronto General Hospital, 3 Eaton North, 200 Elizabeth Street,*
*Toronto, Ontario M5G 2C4, Canada*

Adults with congenital heart disease (CHD) are a considerable challenge to anesthesiologists because of the management they require not only during cardiac surgery but also during noncardiac surgery, acute (postoperative) pain, labor and delivery, and while undergoing conscious sedation for diagnostic and interventional procedures. The adult patient population with CHD includes those with uncorrected, corrected, and palliated congenital heart defects. Patients presenting for repair or revision of a complex congenital heart defect will likely be under the care of an existing CHD team in a tertiary care center [1,2]. The increasing number of adults with CHD mandates the creation of more specialized centers to manage the long term and emergency care of these patients [3–5]. The anesthesiologist is a crucial member of the CHD team. This article addresses the issues that must be considered in establishing anesthetic and perioperative services in a center that provides specialized care for adults with CHD.

Adult patients with CHD have unique adaptive physiologic considerations. They often have a co-existing disease or anatomy with a surgical intervention planned that is in conflict with these considerations, creating management hurdles for the perioperative team. The challenge for the anesthesiologist is to understand the underlying pathophysiology of each CHD patient and to anticipate areas of conflict by tailoring the intraoperative management to minimize the adverse effects the co-existing disease or the operative procedure on the patient's hemodynamics. Several recent reviews are directed toward anesthesia in

this challenging group of patients for cardiac and noncardiac surgery [6–10], as well as reviews in the internal medicine and cardiology literature providing overviews of CHD in adults [1,11–14].

Although much effort has been made to transition the teenager successfully to an adult CHD center, a substantial number of patients are "lost to follow-up" [15]. In addition to managing the patient's perioperative care, the anesthesiologist may have to reunite the patient with a CHD cardiologist. Patients will often minimize the extent of their cardiac disease and focus on the simplest explanation of their problem [16]. In a survey of 1941 adult patients who had CHD and who had been lost to follow-up (> 5 years with no cardiology contact), Wacker [17] found that 96% regarded themselves as healthy and fit, and 68% had no regular medical follow-up.

## Preoperative assessment

The first encounter with the CHD patient is either at the preadmission outpatient consultation or as an inpatient before a surgical procedure or therapeutic intervention. The urgency of the proposed procedure will dictate how much detailed information can be obtained. In emergency situations, such as an acute abdomen or cardioversion, the history will be obtained while preparing to act, and it is imperative that consultant anesthesiologists have knowledge of and experience with CHD or access to colleagues who do either within their own department or by telephone.

An anesthesia consultation includes a discussion of previous surgery and intensive care unit (ICU) admissions. A source of tremendous anxiety for some adult CHD patients is the memory of

E-mail address: jacek.karski@uhn.on.ca (J. Karski).

previous episodes of awareness in the operating room or the ICU [10,18,19]. A review of systems includes questions about asthma, smoking, recreational drugs, alcohol use, renal function, the gastrointestinal tract, endocrine issues, and the presence of and type of a pacemaker, as well as when it was last checked. In all women of childbearing age, the date of the last normal menstrual cycle and the possibility of pregnancy must be considered. In elective cases, extremes of body weight have warranted a delay of surgery for nutritional supplementation or weight loss. Previous anesthetic records and ICU admissions often contain information vital to the anesthetic plan but may not be included in cardiology summaries or dictated surgical notes and may take a few days to procure. The patient's parents may provide much of the history and may need as much reassurance as the patient [16]. It is important to establish good rapport at this time because the anesthesiologist and his or her ICU colleagues will have an intense exposure to the family in the days to come.

It is helpful to have a clear picture of what the patient's innate anatomy was. With this information, the anesthesiologist can follow how surgical intervention has altered the patient's hemodynamics. The blood pressure in both arms should be assessed and the arterial and venous access sites inspected in anticipation of monitoring and resuscitation. Airway assessment and management are critical to the plan for induction and for extubation of the patient. The presence of systemic to pulmonary artery shunts (Blalock-Taussig [BT], Potts, Waterston-Cooley) or a cavopulmonary anastomosis (Glenn or Fontan) is important to note in planning the ventilation and positioning. In a classic BT shunt, the subclavian artery is divided and anastomosed end-to-side to the ipsilateral pulmonary artery. The ipsilateral radial pulse is lost or diminished. Some patients may have had bilateral BT shunts or a BT shunt on one side and arterial cutdowns on the other side. In these patients, monitoring of the central arterial pressure will need to be done from a femoral or high brachial artery. More recent BT shunts may have used a Gore-Tex graft from the intact subclavian to the ipsilateral pulmonary artery. The ipsilateral radial pulse is intact. A Waterston-Cooley shunt is an anastomosis between the posterior aspect of the aorta and the anterior aspect of the right pulmonary artery. A Potts shunt is between the side of the thoracic aorta at the level near the ductus origin and the left pulmonary artery. The superior vena cava

may be connected directly to both pulmonary arteries (bidirectional cavopulmonary) or to the right pulmonary artery (classic Glenn). Long-standing Glenn shunts may be associated with hypoxemia related to pulmonary arteriovenous shunts, as well as systemic venous collaterals [20].

## Pathophysiology of congenital heart disease

### Respiratory issues

Most adults who have CHD have abnormal static lung function when compared with age-matched controls [21]. Although this may have relevance in the recovery room or ICU, it is less likely to influence management of ventilation in the operating room. The ability to increase cardiac output in response to stress is reduced in a wide selection of congenital lesions [22]. Patients may have hypoplastic pulmonary arteries and a diminished number of alveoli related to a previous systemic to pulmonary artery shunt [23]. This difference is a major consideration in positioning the patient in the operating room if the patient's hypoplastic lung is the dependant lung or, worse, the dependent lung in one-lung anesthesia.

### Hypoxemia and shunting

Low oxygen delivery to tissues may be caused by inadequate central oxygenation of blood as occurs in right-to-left shunts. Patients with left-to-right or bidirectional shunts will have decreased delivery of oxygen to the systemic circulation to the extent that pulmonary blood flow exceeds systemic blood flow. The presence of high oxygen saturation does not ensure adequate oxygen delivery. If a patient has a large atrial septal defect (ASD) or common atrium without any outflow tract obstruction, a dramatic fall in pulmonary vascular resistance (PVR) will cause a greater mismatch in blood flow by increasing pulmonary and decreasing systemic circulations. The patient's increased arterial oxygen saturation is at the expense of systemic output; therefore, a pink patient may paradoxically develop a metabolic acidosis. In the management of left-to-right shunts, one should always keep in mind the balance of PVR and systemic vascular resistance (SVR), regardless of the level of the shunt (atrial, ventricular, or great vessels), and choose anesthetic agents and ventilation strategies that will maintain a balance of the PVR and SVR. Residual left-to-right shunts also predispose patients to ventilation perfusion mismatching. There are theoretical delays with inhalational induction in the presence of a right-to-left shunt and in intravenous induction in the presence of a left-to-right shunt, but they have little clinical impact.

Complex cyanotic patients may never have had a palliative surgical procedure but may develop substantial aortopulmonary collaterals. As a result, in addition to an intracardiac right-to-left shunt, these patients have a significant left-to-right shunt through their collaterals. Aortopulmonary collaterals may connect with the central pulmonary arteries or supply a segment of lung independently of the pulmonary circulation. The coronary arteries compete for diastolic blood flow with these aortopulmonary collaterals, and maneuvers that increase the left-to-right shunt compromise myocardial perfusion, putting an increased strain on the systemic ventricle such that it may start to fail and contribute to pulmonary venous hypertension and pulmonary edema [24].

*Hematologic considerations in congenital heart disease*

The hematologic considerations in complex cyanotic heart disease are problematic in any surgery. Oxygen delivery to the tissues depends on many variables, which include the inspired oxygen concentration, minute ventilation, diffusion capacity, cardiac output, tissue extraction, and hemoglobin concentration. The increase in red blood cell mass is an adaptive response to hypoxemia resulting in many cyanotic patients having hematocrits in excess of 70%. There is no agreed upon level of expected hemoglobin for a given degree of hypoxemia, but a patient with a resting saturation under 85% on room air should have a hemoglobin of at least 18. Decompensated erythrocytosis is defined as a high hematocrit with moderate to severe symptoms of hyperviscosity [25]. Iron deficiency is common in cyanotic heart disease and causes red cells to change from flexible biconcave disks to inflexible microspheres. Microcytic iron-deficient erythrocytes have reduced oxygen-carrying capacity and reduced deformability, exacerbating symptoms of hyperviscosity and decreasing oxygen delivery [26]. Preoperative fasting or a bowel preparation may create or exacerbate symptoms of hyperviscosity, and preoperative hydration should be maintained orally or intravenously.

Production of red cells is increased in response to tissue hypoxia but not that of other cell lines or coagulation factors. Tempe and Virmani have published a comprehensive review of coagulation abnormalities in cyanotic heart disease describing thrombocytopenia, platelet function abnormalities, decreased production of coagulation factors, vitamin K deficiency, and primary fibrinolysis [26]. The problem of perioperative coagulopathy in cyanotic heart disease is well known, and adequate transfusion services must exist when contemplating surgery, including labor and delivery.

**Preparing the patient**

To avoid strokes, precautions against air emboli must be taken in all patients with right-to-left shunts, but "air filters" or "bubble traps" are not a substitute for meticulous de-airing of all intravenous lines, stopcocks, and injection ports. Air filters frequently obstruct at the most inopportune times, particularly with propofol, making it difficult to infuse blood through the line. Before connecting the intravenous line to the patient, one should recheck the line because bubbles can mysteriously reappear. When injecting into a line, it is helpful to use a stopcock with the syringe held vertically with the injection port inferior to the syringe. One should aspirate before injection and tap the connector, allowing any air bubbles to float to the superior aspect of the syringe. Nitrous oxide ($N_2O$) may increase PVR and exacerbate an air embolus, and its use is discouraged.

Premedication should be given with the patient's physiology in mind. Knowledge of room air saturation before sedation is also helpful in monitoring the patient in the presurgical waiting area. Patients who are dependent on maintaining a balance of PVR and SVR should wait in a monitored setting. Too much sedation may result in hypercarbia and falling oxygen saturation, whereas an antibiotic such as vancomycin may drastically lower the SVR. In complex cases, the choice of anesthetic agents is not as important as the knowledge and care with which the anesthesiologist manages the patient's hemodynamics.

**Pharmacology of anesthetic agents**

The components of general anesthesia include hypnosis, narcosis, and surgical exposure. The delivery can be intravenously or via volatile anesthetic agents. Conscious sedation involves the use of hypnotics and narcotics in a spontaneously breathing patient and in the past has been referred to as a "neuroleptic technique."

For various reasons, volatile (inhalational) anesthetic agents cause dose-dependent decreases in the systemic blood pressure. Halothane and enflurane cause a dose-dependent decrease in myocardial contractility, whereas isoflurane, sevoflurane, and desflurane cause a decrease in SVR with little effect on cardiac output. All volatile anesthetic agents lower the arrhythmogenic threshold for endogenous and exogenous epinephrine. Halothane has little direct effect on the coronary vasculature, whereas isoflurane, sevoflurane, and desflurane all cause mild coronary vasodilatation. These agents all attenuate the effects of myocardial ischemia, and the subject of ischemic preconditioning is currently a major focus of investigation. The volatile anesthetic agents display variable effects on the pulmonary vasculature including hypoxic pulmonary vasoconstriction. Halothane causes a flow-independent pulmonary vasoconstriction, whereas sevoflurane and desflurane do not alter hypoxic pulmonary vasoconstriction. All volatile anesthetic agents inhibit the baroreceptor reflex [27].

The volatile anesthetic agents are used as a component of general anesthesia, and the agent selected should complement the physiologic goals in the adult patient with CHD. For example, a patient with a cavopulmonary anastomosis will do better with isoflurane than halothane because the cardiac output is maintained, and there is a drop in the SVR while PVR is maintained. Patients with dynamic outflow tract obstruction do well with halothane because it decreases myocardial contractility without dropping the vascular resistance.

Nitrous oxide is an insoluble gas used as an adjunct to general anesthesia and is delivered in conjunction with oxygen in concentrations of 50% to 70%. It is used occasionally in obstetric anesthesia in a concentration of 50% mixed with 50% oxygen when a patient arrives in active or precipitous labor and there is insufficient time for an epidural. Nitrous oxide causes a decrease in venous capacitance, moderate increases in pulmonary arterial pressures, and a mild decrease in contractility, limiting its use in patients who have CHD. Additionally, nitrous oxide diffuses rapidly into closed gas spaces within the body such as the pneumothorax, pneumoperitoneum, and venous air emboli. Alveolar concentrations of 50% to 75% correlate with twofold to fourfold increases in the volume of the gas space. The potential for venous air emboli constitutes an absolute contraindication of nitrous oxide [28].

The intravenous hypnotic agents include propofol, barbiturates (thiopental), benzodiazepines (midazolam), etomidate, and ketamine. Propofol is an alkylphenol that is widely used in anesthesia practice for induction, maintenance of anesthesia, and sedation in the ICU. In healthy patients it causes a significant decrease in the systolic arterial pressure, stroke volume, cardiac index, and SVR. Midazolam is a water soluble benzodiazepine with rapid onset and short duration of action and is cleared significantly faster than diazepam or lorazepam. When used in induction doses of 0.05 to 0.2 mg/kg, it is associated with mild decreases in the mean arterial pressure and heart rate. Midazolam has no analgesic properties and is used routinely in the induction of cardiac patients in conjunction with fentanyl. Thiopental is a barbiturate with a short onset of action, rapid redistribution half-life, but a much longer elimination half-life than midazolam or propofol. It is known to increase venous capacitance, decrease venous return, decrease cardiac index, and increase heart rate. It will significantly decrease cardiovascular parameters in hypovolemic patients and patients with impaired ventricular function. Etomidate is a carboxylated imidazole derivative that is reported to have minimal cardiovascular effects but has been shown to suppress directly adrenal-cortical function. It is not commercially available in the jurisdiction of the author. It appears to have advantages in emergency situations to induce a patient who is hypovolemic or has tamponade. The controversy of the suppression of the stress response has limited the popularity of this drug in anesthesia and intensive care medicine [29]. Ketamine is another agent that has advantages in the unstable and hypovolemic patient but with unpleasant side effects of hallucinations and vivid dreams (nightmares). It is a phencyclidine derivative with profound analgesic properties. In contrast to the other hypnotic agents mentioned, it stimulates the cardiovascular system by the central nervous system, causing increases in heart rate and pulmonary arterial pressure. These effects can be minimized by premedication with benzodiazepines. Ketamine is a direct myocardial depressant [27].

Opioids can be naturally occurring, semisynthetic, or synthetic and act at the opioid receptor to produce a pharmacologic effect. The term *narcotic* is used interchangeably but has a legal implication meaning a controlled substance that can produce dependency and addiction. Examples of naturally occurring opioids are morphine and codeine. Semisynthetics include hydromorphone and meperidine. Synthetics include fentanil, sufentanil, and remifentanil. Morphine is associated with significant hypotension owing to histamine release. Its use in cardiac anesthesia diminished with the advent of synthetic narcotics that have minimal cardiovascular impact [27]. Although there are minimal cardiovascular considerations, opiates are well known to be central respiratory depressants and in the spontaneously breathing patient will raise the apneic threshold (the alveolar carbon dioxide level at which respiration is stimulated) [28].

Neuromuscular blockers are either depolarizing, such as succinylcholine, or nondepolarizing, such as pancuronium and rocuronium. The patient is paralyzed, and the surgeon is provided with sufficient exposure to operate. They have no direct effect on the myocardium and few cardiovascular consequences. Pancuronium may cause a mild tachycardia. The duration of neuromuscular blockade depends on the agent used as well as the hepatic and renal reserve of the patient. These factors must be taken into consideration in planning the postoperative emergence and extubation of the patient.

## Regional anesthesia

Regional anesthesia can include neural axial blocks (epidural and spinal anesthesia) as well as region-specific techniques such as axillary, inguinal, and others. Regional anesthesia is often used in conjunction with general anesthesia and conscious sedation to provide intraoperative and postoperative pain relief. All patients must have a normal coagulation profile. Both spinal and epidural anesthesia cause a significant drop in preload and afterload because the sympathetic nervous system is affected in addition to the sensory and motor blockade. These hemodynamic effects are more pronounced with spinal anesthesia. Absolute contraindications to epidural and spinal anesthesia are local infection at the site of injection, sepsis, and patient refusal.

Epidural anesthesia involves insertion of a catheter into the potential space exterior to the dura. The technique is most commonly used in the lumbar region for relief of pain in labor and for cesarean section. The advantage of an epidural is that local anesthetic and narcotic can be slowly injected to achieve the desired block. Hemodynamic consequences such as a drop in preload

from venodilation and a drop in SVR can be anticipated, particularly with arterial monitoring. Thoracic epidurals are used in conjunction with general anesthesia for management of postoperative pain during upper abdominal and thoracic surgery.

Spinal anesthesia involves a smaller needle advanced across the dura. Local anesthetics and opioids are injected directly into the cerebrospinal fluid. This technique is limited to the lumbar region as the spinal cord ends at L1. Only one dose is administered, and the block has a finite duration. Should the block wear off before the end of the procedure, the patient will likely need conversion to a general anesthetic. The onset of the block is rapid, as are the hemodynamic consequences. The height and distribution of the block can be influenced by altering the density of the local anesthetic solution in relation to the cerebrospinal fluid and positioning of the patient. The duration of the block is dependent on the agent used and whether adrenaline is added to the local anesthetic solution. Spinal anesthesia is widely used in cesarean sections; however, in the adult parturient with CHD, an epidural with a slower onset of action would be desirable. Situations in which spinal anesthesia would be contraindicated would include unrestricted left-to-right shunts (because of the possibility of converting them to right-to-left shunts) and preload-dependent lesions, such as patients with a Fontan circulation, Ebstein's anomaly, tetralogy of Fallot with right ventricular dysfunction, and patients with left-sided outflow tract obstruction.

## Noncardiac surgery

The general considerations for operating on the adult with CHD can be demanding. Noncardiac surgical procedures also pose particular challenges, including one-lung ventilation, jet ventilation for thoracic and tracheal procedures, and procedures that involve insufflation of $CO_2$ into a body cavity. There are also issues related to placing the patient in the lateral, prone, and Trendelenburg positions, and head up for prolonged periods of time. Warner and coworkers [30] retrospectively reviewed the records of 276 adult CHD patients less than 50 years old over a 6-year period and found that patients with cyanosis who received treatment for heart failure and who were in poor general health were at higher risk of complications. This study also found that operations on the respiratory and neurologic systems were associated with high frequencies of complications. Ammash and coworkers [31] retrospectively evaluated 58 adult CHD patients with Eisenmenger syndrome and found that among the 24 patients who underwent noncardiac surgery there were two deaths. One of the deaths followed an appendectomy in a community hospital; the other occurred in a high-risk patient having spinal fusion at a tertiary care center who was in the prone position for an anesthetic time of 525 minutes. Whether CHD patients should be referred to regional tertiary care centers for care by a subspecialist cardiac anesthesiologist or cared for at their local center where their primary cardiologist can follow them is controversial. Many regional cardiac surgical centers do not provide cardiac surgery for adults with CHD but do have cardiac and thoracic trained anesthesiologists and intensive care and blood transfusion facilities that would be able to attend to the situations outlined in the following sections.

## Positioning

### Lateral

In the lateral position, the anesthetized paralyzed patient has a mismatch of ventilation and perfusion. Nephrectomy, thoracotomy, and hip procedures are examples of surgery performed in the lateral position. There is relatively good ventilation and decreased perfusion in the "up" nondependent lung and relatively decreased ventilation but good perfusion in the "down" dependent lung. There is a degree of right-to-left shunt in the "down" dependent lung during two-lung ventilation in the lateral position and a resultant increase in the alveolar arterial oxygen gradient [28]. These factors must be taken into consideration in positioning a patient with pulmonary arteriovenous fistulas and systemic arterial-to-pulmonary arterial shunts, particularly if the shunt has caused hypoplasia of one of the lungs.

### Head up (reverse Trendelenburg)

Head and neck surgery, as well as procedures in the upper abdomen such as cholecystectomy, require the head-up position. The head-up position combined with raised intra-abdominal pressure, laparotomy, and laparoscopic insufflation of $CO_2$ will dramatically reduce preload. In upper abdominal surgery, the abdominal contents or the insufflation of $CO_2$ will push upward against the diaphragm and necessitate higher inspiratory pressures. This factor in combination with the decrease in venous return will compromise preload-dependent right ventricles in patients who have Ebstein's anomaly, tetralogy of Fallot with right ventricular dysfunction, or passive pulmonary perfusion (eg, cavopulmonary anastomosis and Fontan circulations) in whom adequate venous filling pressures and low intrathoracic pressures are needed. In head and neck surgery, central venous monitoring with brachial central lines enables the anesthesiologist to maintain adequate filling pressures. Consideration of conversion of a laparoscopic to an open procedure may be needed in some situations. Cases that involve caval occlusion or compression will necessitate open and frequent communication between the anesthesiologist and the surgeon in addition to central venous monitoring and ventilation strategies to minimize intrathoracic pressure.

### Head down (Trendelenburg)

Gynecologic and urologic procedures involve steep head-down positioning, that is, Trendelenburg and lithotomy, and may be problematic for patients with Glenn shunts, Fontan procedures, and other cavopulmonary anastomoses in which systemic venous hypertension could compromise cerebral perfusion. The abdominal contents are pushed up against the diaphragm, and the patient must be mechanically ventilated with higher inspiratory pressures even though he or she may have difficulty tolerating positive pressure ventilation. If the central venous pressures are high, increasing contractility with an inotrope will improve the cerebral perfusion pressure.

### Prone

The prone or face-down position has physiologic consequences for CHD patients. Once the patient is draped and the case has started, the anesthesiologist will have no access to the precordium or neck and limited access to the airway. Spinal instrumentation is the most common procedure in which the prone position is used, but rectal procedures may also be done prone. Central venous access must be obtained before positioning. There is impaired venous return owing to direct venous compression in the pelvis and subsequent venous pooling in the legs. Compression of the abdominal and thoracic compartments can occur despite the use of a bolster or special frame designed to allow the abdominal compartment to hang free [28]. Cardiopulmonary resuscitation is not possible in the prone position, and a bed (on which to roll the patient) must be kept immediately available should an event occur. Pads for cardioversion can be applied before draping. The series by Ammash and coworkers reported a death in an Eisenmenger patient following spinal surgery in the prone position [31]. A case report of a 14-year-old boy with a Fontan circulation who successfully underwent spinal instrumentation in the prone position highlights these challenges [32].

*One-lung ventilation*

Situations in which one-lung ventilation may be needed would be the placement or extraction of epicardial atrial pacemaker wires, thoracotomy for pulmonary hemorrhage, chylothorax, or lung biopsy, and procedures involving the descending thoracic aorta. Anesthesiologists can ventilate the two lungs independently by means of double-lumen endotracheal tubes, or one lung with the use of bronchial blockers. Once the "up" nondependent lung is not ventilated, there is additional right-to-left shunting because that lung is perfused and not ventilated. Minute alveolar ventilation is increased in the lung that is "down" dependent and able to compensate for carbon dioxide elimination, but there will likely be a further increase in the alveolar arterial oxygen gradient and a drop in the oxygen saturation of the arterial blood [28]. It does not require much imagination to see that this scenario could convert a previous left-to-right shunt to a right-to-left shunt. This situation may be especially difficult in patients who have Eisenmenger syndrome and a high PVR, as well as in Glenn and Fontan circulations where the PVR must be kept as low as possible to fill the left atrium [6,33]. Thoracic surgeons also use a technique of carbon dioxide insufflation into the thoracic cavity referred to as "video-assisted thoracoscopic surgery" where the lung is partially collapsed and, in addition to the mechanical increase in PVR and right-to-left shunt in the nonventilated lung, the arterial carbon dioxide level is elevated from the insufflated carbon dioxide.

*Laparoscopic procedures*

Laparoscopic procedures involve insufflation of carbon dioxide into the peritoneal cavity creating a pneumoperitoneum and are widely used in general, gynecologic, and urologic surgery. The insufflation of $CO_2$ causes a rise in the arterial carbon dioxide concentration owing to vascular absorption across the peritoneum and intravascular embolization. The extent of the cardiovascular changes is primarily dependent on the intra-abdominal pressure attained and the patient's position. This rise in intra-abdominal pressure is transmitted to the chest, causing decreased lung volumes and decreased compliance necessitating increased inflation pressures in mechanically ventilated patients [34]. The head-up position and laparoscopy will reduce venous return, cardiac output, and mean arterial pressure and will increase PVR [35]. Although the patient will have increased intrathoracic pressures, increasing the respiratory rate with smaller tidal volumes and pharmacologic interventions to dilate the pulmonary circulation and improve contractility can overcome the limitations of laparoscopic surgery. If the anesthesiologist is unable to compensate, conversion to an open procedure must be contemplated and the threshold for this decision discussed with the surgeon and attending cardiologist ahead of time.

*Shared airway*

Situations in which the surgeon and the anesthesiologist share the airway involve laryngoscopy and bronchoscopy using the technique of jet ventilation. Tracheal complications of a prolonged ICU stay would be one of the indications for these procedures, and a patient may need evaluation if a complicated cardiac revision is under consideration. In a diagnostic scope, the ventilation can be on 100% oxygen, but if the operation involves laser of the airway, the portion of the procedure using laser must be done on room air to prevent an airway fire. The anesthesiologist delivers intermittent short bursts of pressurized air/oxygen to the airway, and the conventional method of monitoring is observation of arterial blood gases and movement of the chest wall. In between the brief periods of ventilation, while the patient is left apneic so the surgeon can operate on the trachea or larynx, the oxygen saturation will drop and the arterial $CO_2$ will rise. The anesthetic is delivered completely intravenously, and these cases require paralysis and vigilance in monitoring, usually with an arterial line. The nature of the operation compromises the anesthesiologist's ability to ventilate the patient effectively, and there is no way of regulating or monitoring the pressure delivered to the lungs. This situation would be problematic for any patient dependent on a low PVR, such as the patient

578 HEGGIE & KARSKI

with tetralogy with right ventricular dysfunction and pulmonary insufficiency, as well as patients with Fontan circulations. Complications include pneumothorax, pneumomediastinum, and compromise of airway patency.

**Diagnostic and interventional services**

Anesthesiologists are increasingly involved in cardiologic interventional and diagnostic services either as a provider of anesthetic services or as a collaborator in perioperative transesophageal echocardiography (TEE) monitoring in cardiac surgery [36,37]. Anesthesia for diagnostic catheterization or TEE must permit the patient's physiology under anesthesia to reflect his or her awake and ambulatory state as much as possible. Most anesthetic agents lower SVR and lessen the severity of regurgitant lesions. Ketamine is well known to stimulate the central sympathetic nervous system and has been found to counteract the SVR-lowering effects of the hypnotic propofol when the two are used concomitantly. Ketamine has the added advantage of allowing spontaneous breathing on an inspired oxygen concentration close to that of room air. It has the disadvantage of occasionally causing unpleasant or dysphoric dreams when used alone [38,39].

The same considerations would apply to anesthesia for TEE, because the goal is not to alter the patient's ambulatory physiology. These procedures are performed most easily with the patient in the lateral position and breathing spontaneously after the oropharynx has been sprayed with topical lidocaine. Appropriate recovery facilities must be available, and it is safer to conduct these studies in a monitored facility, operating room, post anesthetic recovery room, or coronary care unit, particularly if the indication for TEE is to rule out thrombus before cardioversion. The cardioversion can be performed immediately following the procedure, before emergence from anesthesia, with the patient in the lateral position as the airway is unprotected owing to the topical local anesthetic. In an operating room or ICU setting, any complications related to the cardioversion can be addressed quickly because the appropriate staff and equipment are immediately available.

In interventional cases, the diagnosis has been established, the cardiologist must be able to conduct the procedure safely without distraction, and the patient must be free of pain [36]. Examples would include stenting of coarctation,

percutaneous valve insertion, insertion of biventricular pacing leads, and ablation therapy. Interventional cases necessitate a deeper level of conscious sedation or general anesthesia and possible neuromuscular blockade [37]. When diagnostic angiography precedes the intervention, it is reasonable to use conscious sedation as outlined previously and convert to a general anesthetic for the intervention. Recovery of the patient is best served in the post anesthetic care unit or a monitored ICU setting not only for hemodynamic monitoring but also because the degree of somnolence and the risk of incomplete reversal of a neuromuscular blockade may exceed the capabilities of the recovery area of the interventional suite [37].

**Arrhythmias and cardioversions**

Arrhythmias are common in adult patients with CHD. In a large survey of adults with CHD, Kaemmerer and colleagues demonstrated that one fourth of all admissions to a specialized adult CHD facility were urgent and unscheduled. The most common reason for readmission was cardiovascular, of which arrhythmia was the most common [4]. A cross-sectional study of 2609 adults with CHD found that sudden death was the most common cause of death (26%) [40]. Ventricular arrhythmias occur more commonly in patients with left-sided obstruction, tetralogy of Fallot, and severe ventricular dysfunction [41]. The Euro Heart Survey program published a retrospective cohort study performed from 1998 to April 2004 of more than 4000 adult patients with one of eight different congenital heart diagnoses. The incidence of supraventricular arrhythmias was 18% overall and highest in the Fontan group (45%), followed by secundum ASD (28%), transposition (26%), and tetralogy of Fallot (20%). The incidence of ventricular arrhythmias was 5% overall and highest in the tetralogy of Fallot group (14%) [3].

Anesthesia for cardioversion is a simple and uncomplicated procedure that requires a short hypnotic agent, support of the airway, and ventilation for a brief period of time. Nevertheless, cardioversions are fraught with complications, and the anesthesiologist must anticipate these complications and have a clear back up plan in mind before proceeding. A telephone consultation with a cardiovascular anesthesiologist experienced with CHD may be warranted. The procedure should take place in a monitored environment that is accessible to ancillary personnel. Should the procedure result in a bradyarrhythmia, the means to pace should be available. This treatment may be via a temporary wire via central venous access or may be performed transcutaneously in the patient who has a cavopulmonary anastomosis (as there will be no intravenous access from above to the ventricle). The procedure may be preceded by TEE to rule out atrial thrombus. Of 52 adults undergoing the Fontan operation, 17 (33%) had asymptomatic thrombi in the right atrium and one in the left atrium, surprisingly with no correlation to the presence of arrhythmias [42]. The considerations for pacemaker insertion as well as defibrillator implant are much like those outlined in preparing for noncardiac surgery but with the additional concerns outlined previously.

## Labor and delivery

Women with CHD comprise the majority of cardiac patients presenting for labor and delivery. These patients are best managed in a high-risk pregnancy unit by a multidisciplinary team from obstetrics, cardiology, anesthesia, and neonatology [43]. Comprehensive reviews of pregnancy and heart disease are in the recent literature, including didactic accounts of the normal cardiovascular changes of pregnancy and the implications for patients with specific congenital heart defects [44–47]. A large prospective multi-center study of 562 pregnant women with cardiac disease (74% with CHD) with 599 pregnancies defined four predictors of primary cardiac events: (1) a prior cardiac event or arrhythmia, (2) a baseline New York Heart Association classification of heart disease greater than II or cyanosis, (3) left-sided heart obstruction, and (4) reduced systemic ventricular function. There was no association between the type of delivery, vaginal versus cesarean section, and peripartum cardiac events [48]. Another study reviewed the records of 90 pregnancies in 53 women with CHD using the same definitions of obstetric, neonatal, and cardiac events as in the previous study and found a cardiac event rate of 19%, of which congestive heart failure was the most common followed by arrhythmias. Independent risk factors for pulmonary edema included a history of congestive heart failure, smoking, and a decreased subpulmonary ejection fraction. All but one of the patients in this study received an epidural [49].

A team conference with anesthesia in attendance should be held early in the patient's pregnancy to plan and disseminate the treatment goals. Epidurals are desirable in most patients, although anticoagulants will preclude this if not stopped in sufficient time. Although there are congenital defects in which any drop in afterload must be avoided, low concentrations of local anesthetics and the use of intrathecal and epidural narcotics will diminish this risk, particularly if initiated slowly with appropriate monitoring and vasopressors available. The extent of invasive monitoring will be dictated by the patient's functional class and type of defect. Central venous and especially pulmonary arterial monitoring should only be used when the information is essential and cannot be obtained any other way. In a patient with a significant aortic coarctation, arterial monitoring below the obstruction is necessary to ascertain the placental perfusion pressure; the proximal aortic pressure may not drop significantly with a low thoracic level epidural, but the distal aortic pressure may drop significantly [50]. The use of nitrates in managing pulmonary hypertension will adversely affect the uterine tone. There are limited reasons to avoid vaginal delivery. The only cardiac indications for cesarean section are Marfan syndrome with a dilated aortic root and the failure to stop warfarin in sufficient time before labor [43].

## Perioperative transesophageal echocardiography

Institutions vary as to whether anesthesiologists or cardiologists provide perioperative TEE monitoring. Who is best suited to do this is subject to debate. Regardless of the primary specialty, the TEE echocardiographer must have additional training in the reading of complex congenital echocardiography [51,52]. The echocardiographer should function independently from the role of the primary anesthesiologist and should be available to return to monitor the patient. Ideally, a collaborative relationship between the cardiology service and the anesthesiology service will exist. An exhaustive TEE review in the adult CHD patient has been published recently by Russell and coworkers [53].

## Cardiac surgery

Patients presenting for repair of a complex congenital anomaly or revision of a previous repair will do so to an established congenital cardiac surgical center, whether pediatric or adult in focus. The acuity of these procedures is much greater than the situations outlined previously, and co-existing disease, particularly respiratory, renal, and hepatic, may disqualify some patients for cardiac surgery. Adults of small stature will have considerations independent of their cardiac anatomy and may require smaller priming volumes for the heart lung machine, a prudent choice of central venous catheters, airway considerations, and vigilance in the administration of parenteral fluids. Large bore intravenous lines with the capability to transfuse fluids at high flow rates are routine, and care must be taken that a "runaway liter" is not inadvertently administered. The adult CHD patient of small stature and compromised ventricular function may not tolerate such a volume load. Precautions for repeat sternotomy include blood readily available for transfusion, heparinization before sternotomy, the use of antifibrinolytics, and access to femoral vessels for cannulation (true for all patients requiring repeat sternotomy). Anesthetic considerations for cardiac surgery in each individual congenital heart defect, beyond the issues outlined herein, are beyond the scope of this article. The adult with CHD is a core topic of a didactic cardiac anesthesia fellowship, but not all graduates will necessarily be involved in the care of these patients. The following discussion presents a brief overview of issues that the cardiac anesthesiologist will encounter and provides an overview for cardiologists participating in the perioperative care of these patients. Several recent reviews detail the management of cardiac anesthesia for this population as well as anesthetic management of specific defects [6,7,10,54,55].

The ICU should be in close proximity to the operating room, and transport should occur in a seamless and monitored fashion. On arrival to the ICU, there must be a surgical and anesthesia report to the nursing, respiratory, and medical staff. Hemodynamic goals and respiratory parameters should be clearly outlined, and a sketch or drawing of the patient's preoperative and postoperative anatomy is helpful. Much of what occurs in the ICU is a natural extension of the anesthetic management in the operating room, and in difficult cases the ICU staff should be available to the operating room to participate in the post bypass care and the determination of goals of care. Once the patient is admitted to the ICU, the attending cardiologist should be involved on a daily basis even though the patient may be under the care of the attending surgeons

and attending ICU physicians. CHD cardiologists can contribute to the postoperative management of arrhythmias, echocardiography interpretation, and interventional consultations. Knowledge of the ICU events will also be helpful in managing the patient on transfer to the ward setting.

*Atrial septal defect, ventricular septal defects, atrioventricular septal defects, and patent ductus arteriosus*

Most cases of secundum ASD and patent ductus arteriosus (PDA) can be closed in the catheterization laboratory with a device [56]. Some ventricular septal defects (VSD) can be managed in the interventional suite [57]. Rarely, patients will need to be transported to the operating room for retrieval of a malpositioned or embolized device. On the rare occasions when a device has embolized, the immediate anesthesia goal is to prevent further travel.

Regardless of the location of the septal defect or the presence of a PDA and the type of closure, there are some basic considerations for the cardiac anesthesiologist as outlined in the anesthesia of patients with left-to-right shunts.

Patients who have their defects closed surgically are likely to have additional cardiac anomalies or have been referred for a Maze procedure to treat atrial arrhythmias. These patients are likely to be older and may also have significant coronary artery disease [58]. Patients who have mitral regurgitation in association with a primum ASD may have pulmonary hypertension that may not be entirely due to increased pulmonary blood flow [59]. Precautions for maintaining an optimal PVR should be observed as outlined previously. Pulmonary vasodilators may be needed post bypass in addition to maintaining an alkalotic pH and ventilating the patient at tidal volumes close to functional residual capacity with minimal airway pressures. Most patients successfully wean from bypass without intravenous nitrates or milrinone, but these agents may be necessary. Occasionally, one will have to add inhalational nitric oxide [60]. A method of portable nitric oxide delivery is essential for leaving the operating room and delivering the patient to the ICU.

*Tetralogy of Fallot*

It is unusual to see an adult with uncorrected tetralogy of Fallot, although this does occur in immigrants whose anatomy was favorable for long-term survival or who originated from a country where surgical intervention was not available [61–63]. Anesthesia for an uncorrected tetralogy of Fallot is well described in Lake's text of congenital heart anesthesia [64]. The most common reasons for reoperation in adults with tetralogy of Fallot corrected in childhood are to repair the right ventricular outflow tract or replace the regurgitant pulmonary valve, to repair a VSD patch leak, or to′ repair severe tricuspid regurgitation [65]. Anesthetic and ICU management must anticipate right ventricular dysfunction, and measures to minimize PVR post bypass and to improve contractility may be indicated, although these patients usually do very well [66]. The use of a pulmonary arterial catheter is unnecessary. Postoperative management should take into account keeping the central venous pressure high as well as maintaining a low PVR with a mild respiratory alkalosis and avoiding extremes of lung volumes. Left ventricular dysfunction will impact negatively on the right ventricular output and should be managed with inotropes and afterload reduction. Arrhythmias should be anticipated and treated preoperatively in the electrophysiology suite or intraoperatively with cryoablation. Patients in whom severe tricuspid regurgitation was an issue preoperatively may need management of a coagulopathy secondary to hepatic congestion.

## Ebstein's anomaly

Ebstein's anomaly is characterized by adherence of one or more tricuspid leaflets to the underlying myocardium with apical displacement of the leaflets, "atrialization" of the right ventricle and a dilated right atrium, and tricuspid regurgitation. Many patients have an ASD that is often associated with a right-to-left shunt. Surgery may include closure of the atrial defect, performance of an antiarrhythmic procedure, reduction of the right atrium, and repair or replacement of the tricuspid valve [67]. Pre-bypass considerations must account for the right-to-left shunt as well as the severe tricuspid regurgitation. Post bypass one should anticipate right ventricular dysfunction and take measures to optimize contractility and reduce the afterload of the right ventricle [68]. Pulmonary vasodilators such as milrinone or inhalational nitric oxide used with inotropes such as dobutamine may be needed in the postbypass period. Chronic hepatic congestion from severe tricuspid regurgitation may affect the severity of postoperative coagulation.

## Transposition of the great arteries with a Mustard or Senning procedure

Adults with a transposition of the great arteries usually have had an atrial type of repair (Mustard or Senning operation) as a young child. This operation leaves the patient with the morphologic right ventricle as the systemic ventricle and the tricuspid valve as the systemic atrioventricular valve, both of which may fail in adult life. Complications also include baffle leaks, superior vena cava obstruction, inferior vena cava obstruction, pulmonary venous obstruction, and arrhythmias (sinus node, atrial, or ventricular). These patients seldom present for cardiac reoperation but may present for pacemaker insertion or other surgical procedures. Anesthetic management of systemic ventricular (right ventricular) failure in a Mustard patient is much like managing a patient with a dilated cardiomyopathy. Central venous monitoring in the Mustard patient can be problematic. A pulmonary artery catheter or pacing wire must traverse the intra-atrial baffle to get to the morphologic left ventricle in the subpulmonary position. There is the potential for inducing arrhythmia. The pulmonary arterial catheter will appear to make a sharp "hairpin" turn or loop as it enters the pulmonary artery from the morphologic left ventricle. The morphologic right ventricle (systemic ventricle) often becomes dilated and hypokinetic. Anesthetic agents with minimal effects on contractility that lower SVR are desirable.

## Transposition of the great arteries with pulmonary stenosis and a Rastelli procedure

Transposition of the great arteries may be associated with a VSD and pulmonary stenosis. The Rastelli procedure redirects blood flow from the left ventricle to the aorta at the ventricular level, and a valved extracardiac conduit is placed from the right ventricle to the pulmonary artery. These patients frequently present for reoperation because of obstruction of the extracardiac conduit. The right ventricle to pulmonary artery conduit lies just beneath the sternum and is vulnerable to external compression, as well as trauma or laceration on re-entering the chest. Occasionally, the conduit is critically narrowed, and all monitoring lines as well as femoral cannulation and heparinization are performed before induction and endotracheal intubation performed with ensuing positive pressure ventilation. Spontaneously breathing intravenous conscious sedation with propofol and ketamine mixtures are effective. Adequate venous return and filling pressures must be maintained, and anesthetic agents that lower preload by causing venodilation must be avoided.

### Congenitally corrected (left) transposition of the great arteries

Congenitally corrected transposition of the great arteries requires discordant atrioventricular and ventriculoarterial connections. The circulation is physiologically viable, but the morphologic right ventricle is, from birth, the systemic ventricle. Such patients may present for systemic tricuspid valve replacement, for replacement of the previously placed valved conduit, or for correction of a VSD and pulmonary stenosis in a fashion similar to that of the Rastelli procedure. The anesthetic management is similar to that for a dilated cardiomyopathy, as described in the section on Mustard patients. Patients may present with systemic ventricular dysfunction, systemic atrioventricular valve regurgitation, or atrioventricular block [69]. The associated lesions or complications usually dictate the patient's operative and anesthetic care.

### Glenn and Fontan operations

Single ventricle physiology is treated by bypassing the right side of the heart by direct connection of the inferior vena cava or superior vena cava to the pulmonary arteries using a bidirectional cavopulmonary shunt or the Fontan operation (complete nonpulsatile systemic venous return to the pulmonary artery). The superior vena cava may be connected directly to both pulmonary arteries (bidirectional cavopulmonary) or to the right pulmonary artery only (classic Glenn operation). A cavopulmonary shunt may be a stage on the path to a Fontan operation. Fontan described a total right-sided heart bypass that has been subject to numerous modifications over the years [70–74]. Although the differences in anatomy may not change one's approach to maintaining the physiology, the anatomic differences in these modifications may influence central venous monitoring. In a patient with a classic Glenn operation, a jugular or subclavian venous catheter will not reach the heart, nor will it in a bidirectional Glenn operation if the superior vena cava has been divided from the right atrium. The

pressure in these central venous catheters reflects the pulmonary arterial pressure in the involved lung.

Most adult patients will present for a Maze procedure and revision of a previous Fontan operation [74,75]. The anesthetic care of this group of patients is among the most challenging in an adult cardiac anesthesia practice. It is important to know if the Fontan anastomosis is fenestrated, with a right-to-left shunt. Precautions for venous air emboli must be taken. Fontan patients are highly dependent upon adequate preload. Pulmonary blood flow is dependent upon the gradient between the vena cava and the left atrium; therefore, increased PVR (induced by hypoxia, hypercapnia, light anesthesia, increased/decreased extremes in lung volumes) will have deleterious effects. The pre-bypass goals are no different than post bypass. For patients to thrive, they must have a controlled regular rhythm (preferably sinus), sufficient right-sided filling pressures, minimal PVR, a competent systemic atrioventricular valve, maintained left ventricular function, and afterload reduction for the left ventricle. The only means to monitor left atrial filling pressure in these patients is by using a left atrial line. The gradient between the right-sided filling pressures and the left atrial line (transpulmonary pressure) should be above 10 mm Hg, and colloids including blood products are administered if left atrial pressures are less than 8 mm Hg or transpulmonary pressures less than 8 mm Hg. Gradients of more than 2 to 3 mm Hg can be clinically significant, and confirmation by echo or cardiac catheterization is warranted. Methods to lower or optimize the PVR include hyperventilation and administration of bicarbonate for a pH greater than 7.50, an increase in the inspired concentration of oxygen, optimization of ventilation with appropriate sedation and paralysis if needed, and pulmonary vasodilators both intravenous and inhalational (milrinone, nitrates, prostacyclin, nitric oxide). Atrial pacing or sequential atrioventricular pacing at a higher rate, inotropes to improve contractility, and afterload reduction will all help to improve the cardiac output of the single ventricle.

Coagulopathy is a major issue. Once hemostasis is obtained, ventilation is weaned, preferably with pressure support, and early extubation is the goal. It is prudent to supervise extubation of the patient, because prolonged Valsalva breaths, retching, or coughing against the ventilator may precipitate hemodynamic instability. Problems with pleural effusions and ascites may arise and interfere with ventilation and should be treated promptly with chest drains and peritoneal catheters. In patients with acute renal insufficiency requiring renal replacement therapy, the insertion of the vascular access line must be done with caution because these lines are of relatively wide diameter and may enter or partially occlude the Glenn shunt. Arrhythmias are poorly tolerated, and aggressive attempts to convert to sinus rhythm should be contemplated with the advice of the patient's CHD cardiologist. Hypercoagulability is another issue, and anticoagulation and mechanical factors are indicated to prevent deep venous thrombosis. The optimal type or duration of anticoagulation is not clear [42,76,77].

## Summary

Anesthesia for adults with CHD has many challenging physiologic considerations. Collaborative relationships of a multidisciplinary team including cardiology, cardiac surgery, anesthesiology, and intensive care are essential to ensure positive outcomes in this population for noncardiac and cardiac surgery.

## Acknowledgments

The author thanks Dr. Gary Webb and Dr. William Williams for their encouragement and leadership.

## References

[1] Niwa K, Perloff JK, Webb GD, et al. Survey of specialized tertiary care facilities for adults with congenital heart disease. Int J Cardiol 2004;96(2): 211–6.

[2] Warnes CA, Liberthson R, Danielson GK, et al. Task force 1: the changing profile of congenital heart disease in adult life. J Am Coll Cardiol 2001;37(5): 1170–5.

[3] Engelfriet P, Boersma E, Oechslin E, et al. The spectrum of adult congenital heart disease in Europe: morbidity and mortality in a 5 year follow-up period. The Euro Heart Survey on adult congenital heart disease. Eur Heart J 2005;26(21):2325–33.

[4] Kaemmerer H, Fratz S, Bauer U, et al. Emergency hospital admissions and three-year survival of adults with and without cardiovascular surgery for congenital cardiac disease. J Thorac Cardiovasc Surg 2003; 126(4):1048–52.

[5] Therrien J, Gatzoulis M, Graham T, et al. Canadian Cardiovascular Society Consensus Conference 2001

update: Recommendations for the Management of Adults with Congenital Heart Disease–Part II. Can J Cardiol 2001;17(10):1029–50.

[6] Lovell AT. Anaesthetic implications of grown-up congenital heart disease. Br J Anaesth 2004;93(1): 129–39.

[7] Stayer SA, Andropoulos DB, Russell IA. Anesthetic management of the adult patient with congenital heart disease. Anesthesiol Clin North Am 2003; 21(3):653–73.

[8] Findlow D, Doyle E. Congenital heart disease in adults. Br J Anaesth 1997;78(4):416–30.

[9] Galli KK, Myers LB, Nicolson SC. Anesthesia for adult patients with congenital heart disease undergoing noncardiac surgery. Int Anesthesiol Clin 2001; 39(4):43–71.

[10] Heggie J, Poirier N, Williams W, et al. Anesthetic considerations for adult cardiac surgery patients with congenital heart disease. Semin Cardiothorac Vasc Anesth 2003;7(2):141–52.

[11] Webb G. Improving the care of Canadian adults with congenital heart disease. Can J Cardiol 2005; 21(10):833–8.

[12] Gatzoulis MA. Adult congenital heart disease: education, education, education. Nat Clin Pract Cardiovasc Med 2006;3(1):2–3.

[13] Brickner ME, Hillis LD, Lange RA. Congenital heart disease in adults: first of two parts. N Engl J Med 2000;342(4):256–63.

[14] Brickner ME, Hillis LD, Lange RA. Congenital heart disease in adults: second of two parts. N Engl J Med 2000;342(5):334–42.

[15] Reid GJ, Irvine MJ, McCrindle BW, et al. Prevalence and correlates of successful transfer from pediatric to adult health care among a cohort of young adults with complex congenital heart defects. Pediatrics 2004;113(3):197–205.

[16] Walker F. Precious adults: a lesson in grown-up congenital heart disease. Lancet 2003;362(9379): 241.

[17] Wacker AE. Outcome of operated and unoperated adults with congenital cardiac disease lost to follow-up for more than five years. Am J Cardiol 2005;95:776–9.

[18] Curtis S, Stuart G. Outcome in congenital heart disease. Curr Paediatr 2005;15:549–56.

[19] Tempe DK, Siddiquie RA. Awareness during cardiac surgery. J Cardiothorac Vasc Anesth 1999; 13(2):214–9.

[20] Magee AG, McCrindle BW, Mawson J, et al. Systemic venous collateral development after the bidirectional cavopulmonary anastomosis: prevalence and predictors. J Am Coll Cardiol 1998; 32(2):502–8.

[21] Rigolin VH, Li JS, Hanson MW, et al. Role of right ventricular and pulmonary functional abnormalities in limiting exercise capacity in adults with congenital heart disease. Am J Cardiol 1997;80(3): 315–22.

[22] Fredriksen PM, Veldtman G, Hechter S, et al. Aerobic capacity in adults with various congenital heart diseases. Am J Cardiol 2001;87(3):310–4.

[23] Godart F, Qureshi SA, Simha A, et al. Effects of modified and classic Blalock-Taussig shunts on the pulmonary arterial tree. Ann Thorac Surg 1998; 66(2):512–7.

[24] Fabre OH, Porte HL, Godart FR, et al. Long-term cardiovascular consequences of undiagnosed intra-lobar pulmonary sequestration. Ann Thorac Surg 1998;65(4):1144–6.

[25] Oechslin E. Hematological management of the cyanotic adult with congenital heart disease. Int J Cardiol 2004;97(Suppl):1109–15.

[26] Tempe DK, Virmani S. Coagulation abnormalities in patients with cyanotic congenital heart disease. J Cardiothorac Vasc Anesth 2002;16(6): 752–65.

[27] Grogan K, Nyhan D, Berkowitz D. Pharmacology of anesthetic drugs. In: Kaplan RLK, editor. Kaplan's cardiac anesthesia. 5th edition. Philadelphia: WB Saunders; 2006. p. 165–212.

[28] Miller R. Anesthesia. New York: Churchill Livingstone; 2005.

[29] Jackson WL Jr. Should we use etomidate as an induction agent for endotracheal intubation in patients with septic shock? A critical appraisal. Chest 2005;127(3):1031–8.

[30] Warner MA, Lunn RJ, O'Leary PW, et al. Outcomes of noncardiac surgical procedures in children and adults with congenital heart disease: Mayo Perioperative Outcomes Group. Mayo Clin Proc 1998; 73(8):728–34.

[31] Ammash NM, Connolly HM, Abel MD, et al. Noncardiac surgery in Eisenmenger syndrome. J Am Coll Cardiol 1999;33(1):222–7.

[32] Vischoff D, Fortier LP, Villeneuve E, et al. Anaesthetic management of an adolescent for scoliosis surgery with a Fontan circulation. Paediatr Anaesth 2001;11(5):607–10.

[33] Heller AR, Litz RJ, Koch T. A fine balance—one-lung ventilation in a patient with Eisenmenger syndrome. Br J Anaesth 2004;92(4):587–90.

[34] Gerges JG, Ghassan EK, Jabbour-Khoury SI. Anesthesia for laparoscopy: a review. J Clin Anesth 2006; 18:67–78.

[35] Gutt C, Mehrabi A, Schemmer P, et al. Circulatory and respiratory complications of carbon dioxide insufflation. Dig Surg 2004;21(2):95–105.

[36] Andropoulos DB, Stayer SA. An anesthesiologist for all pediatric cardiac catheterizations: luxury or necessity? J Cardiothorac Vasc Anesth 2003;17(6): 683–5.

[37] Chessa M, Carrozza C, Butera G, et al. The impact of interventional cardiology for the management of adults with congenital heart disease. Catheter Cardiovasc Interv 2006;67:258–64.

[38] Oklu E, Bulutcu FS, Yalcin Y, et al. Which anesthetic agent alters the hemodynamic status during

pediatric catheterization? Comparison of propofol versus ketamine. J Cardiothorac Vasc Anesth 2003;17(6):686–90.

[39] Kogan A, Efrat R, Katz J, et al. Propofol-ketamine mixture for anesthesia in pediatric patients undergoing cardiac catheterization. J Cardiothorac Vasc Anesth 2003;17(6):691–3.

[40] Oechslin EN, Harrison DA, Connelly MS, et al. Mode of death in adults with congenital heart disease. Am J Cardiol 2000;86(10):1111–6.

[41] Khairy P, Dore A, Talajic M, et al. Arrhythmias in adult congenital heart disease. Future drugs—expert review of cardiovascular therapy 2006;4(1):1–32.

[42] Balling G, Vogt M, Kaemmerer H, et al. Intracardiac thrombus formation after the Fontan operation. J Thorac Cardiovasc Surg 2000;119(4):745–52.

[43] Siu S, Coleman J. Heart disease and pregnancy. Heart 2001;85:710–5.

[44] van Mook WN, Peeters L. Severe cardiac disease in pregnancy. Part I. Hemodynamic changes and complaints during pregnancy, and general management of cardiac disease in pregnancy. Curr Opin Crit Care 2005;11(5):430–4.

[45] van Mook WN, Peeters L. Severe cardiac disease in pregnancy. Part II. Impact of congenital and acquired cardiac diseases during pregnancy. Curr Opin Crit Care 2005;11(5):435–48.

[46] Colman J, Siu S. Pregnancy in adult patients with congenital heart disease. Prog Pediatr Cardiol 2003;17:53–60.

[47] Koos BJ. Management of uncorrected, palliated, and repaired cyanotic congenital heart disease in pregnancy. Prog Pediatr Cardiol 2004;19:25–45.

[48] Siu SC, Sermer M, Colman JM, et al. Prospective multicenter study of pregnancy outcomes in women with heart disease. Circulation 2001;104(5):515–21.

[49] Khairy P, Ouyang DW, Fernandes SM, et al. Pregnancy outcomes in women with congenital heart disease. Circulation 2006;113(4):517–24.

[50] Walker E, Malins AF. Anaesthetic management of aortic coarctation in pregnancy. Int J Obstet Anesth 2004;13(4):266–70.

[51] Moran AM, Geva T. Con: pediatric anesthesiologists should not be the primary echocardiographers for pediatric patients undergoing cardiac surgical procedures. J Cardiothorac Vasc Anesth 2001; 15(3):391–3.

[52] Sangwan S, Au C, Mahajan A. Pro: pediatric anesthesiologists should be the primary echocardiographers for pediatric patients undergoing cardiac surgical procedures. J Cardiothorac Vasc Anesth 2001;15(3):388–90.

[53] Russell IA, Rouine-Rapp K, Stratmann G, et al. Congenital heart disease in the adult: a review with Internet-accessible transesophageal echocardiographic images. Anesth Analg 2006;102(3): 694–723.

[54] Andropoulos DB, Stayer SA, Skjonsby BS, et al. Anesthetic and perioperative outcome of teenagers

and adults with congenital heart disease. J Cardiothorac Vasc Anesth 2002;16(6):731–6.

[55] Akpek EA, Miller-Hance WC, Stayer SA, et al. Anesthetic management and outcome of complex late arterial-switch operations for patients with transposition of the great arteries and a systemic right ventricle. J Cardiothorac Vasc Anesth 2005; 19(3):322–8.

[56] Chessa M, Carminati M, Butera G, et al. Early and late complications associated with transcatheter occlusion of secundum atrial septal defect. J Am Coll Cardiol 2002;39(6):1061–5.

[57] Carminati M, Butera G, Chessa M, et al. Transcatheter closure of congenital ventricular septal defect with Amplatzer septal occluders. Am J Cardiol 2005;96(12A):52L–8L.

[58] Gatzoulis MA, Freeman MA, Siu SC, et al. Atrial arrhythmia after surgical closure of atrial septal defects in adults. N Engl J Med 1999;340(11): 839–46.

[59] Gatzoulis MA, Hechter S, Webb GD, et al. Surgery for partial atrioventricular septal defect in the adult. Ann Thorac Surg 1999;67(2):504–10.

[60] Budts W, Van PN, Gillyns H, et al. Residual pulmonary vasoreactivity to inhaled nitric oxide in patients with severe obstructive pulmonary hypertension and Eisenmenger syndrome. Heart 2001;86(5):553–8.

[61] Morton BC, Morch JE, Williams WG. Primary repair of Fallot's tetralogy in an older adult: a 20-year follow-up. Can J Cardiol 1996;12(12): 1268–70.

[62] Presbitero P, Prever SB, Contrafatto I, et al. As originally published in 1988: results of total correction of tetralogy of Fallot performed in adults. Updated in 1996. Ann Thorac Surg 1996;61(6):1870–3.

[63] Hughes CF, Lim YC, Cartmill TB, et al. Total intracardiac repair for tetralogy of Fallot in adults. Ann Thorac Surg 1987;43(6):634–8.

[64] Lake C, Booker P. Pediatric cardiac anesthesia. Philadelphia: Lippincott Williams & Wilkins; 2004.

[65] Oechslin EN, Harrison DA, Harris L, et al. Reoperation in adults with repair of tetralogy of Fallot: indications and outcomes. J Thorac Cardiovasc Surg 1999;118(2):245–51.

[66] Gatzoulis MA, Elliott JT, Guru V, et al. Right and left ventricular systolic function late after repair of tetralogy of Fallot. Am J Cardiol 2000;86(12): 1352–7.

[67] Dearani JA, Danielson GK. Surgical management of Ebstein's anomaly in the adult. Semin Thorac Cardiovasc Surg 2005;17(2):148–54.

[68] Lerner A, Dinardo JA, Comunale ME. Anesthetic management for repair of Ebstein's anomaly. J Cardiothorac Vasc Anesth 2003;17(2):232–5.

[69] Connelly MS, Liu PP, Williams WG, et al. Congenitally corrected transposition of the great arteries in the adult: functional status and complications. J Am Coll Cardiol 1996;27(5):1238–43.

[70] Fontan F, Baudet E. Surgical repair of tricuspid atresia. Thorax 1971;26(3):240–8.

[71] Mavroudis C, Zales VR, Backer CL, et al. Fenestrated Fontan with delayed catheter closure: effects of volume loading and baffle fenestration on cardiac index and oxygen delivery. Circulation 1992;86(5 Suppl):II85–92.

[72] Kreutzer J, Keane JF, Lock JE, et al. Conversion of modified Fontan procedure to lateral atrial tunnel cavopulmonary anastomosis. J Thorac Cardiovasc Surg 1996;111(6):1169–76.

[73] Mavroudis C, Backer CL, Deal BJ, et al. Fontan conversion to cavopulmonary connection and arrhythmia circuit cryoablation. J Thorac Cardiovasc Surg 1998;115(3):547–56.

[74] Mavroudis C, Backer CL, Deal BJ, et al. Total cavopulmonary conversion and maze procedure for patients with failure of the Fontan operation. J Thorac Cardiovasc Surg 2001;122(5):863–71.

[75] van den Bosch AE, Roos-Hesselink JW, Van DR, et al. Long-term outcome and quality of life in adult patients after the Fontan operation. Am J Cardiol 2004;93(9):1141–5.

[76] Walker HA, Gatzoulis MA. Prophylactic anticoagulation following the Fontan operation. Heart 2005; 91(7):854–6.

[77] Monagle P, Karl TR. Thromboembolic problems after the Fontan operation. Semin Thorac Cardiovasc Surg Pediatr Cardiol Surg Annu 2002;5: 36–47.

ELSEVIER
SAUNDERS

Cardiol Clin 24 (2006) 587–605

CARDIOLOGY
CLINICS

# The Team Approach to Pregnancy and Congenital Heart Disease

Henryk Kafka, MD, FRCPC, FACC[a,b,*], Mark R. Johnson, PhD, MRCP, MRCOG[c], Michael A. Gatzoulis, MD, PhD, FACC[a]

[a]Adult Congenital Heart Disease Centre, Royal Brompton Hospital, Sydney Street, London SW3 6NP, UK
[b]Division of Cardiology, Queen's University Cardiovascular Laboratory, Kingston General Hospital, 76 Stewart Street, Kingston, ON, Canada K7L2V7
[c]Academic Obstetrics and Gynaecology, Chelsea and Westminster, 369 Fulham Road, London SW10 9NH, UK

The adult cardiologist is being called upon to see an increasing number of patients who have congenital heart disease. The incidence of this most common inborn defect is generally estimated at 0.8% of all births [1,2]. The advances in pediatric cardiology and surgery have resulted in a marked improvement in survival. Fifty years ago, only 25% of infants who had congenital heart disease (CHD) would survive their first year and now we expect about 85% to survive into adulthood [3]. There are no firm figures as to the real size of this adult population but it is estimated at 800,000 adult patients who have CHD in the United States. With an annual birth rate of 4 million [4], the United States will add another 28,000 infants who have CHD each year, with about 24,000 of these surviving into adulthood and joining the ever-growing list of adults who have congenital heart disease. Survival into adulthood certainly does not equate with cure of their congenital lesions [3,5] and they continue to face medical, surgical, and psychosocial obstacles [5–8]. Among these, some of the most challenging revolve

around sexual function, reproductive issues, and pregnancy [9–11].

In the face of the improved survival among those who have congenital cardiac lesions and with the decreasing incidence of rheumatic heart disease, CHD is now the most common structural cardiac problem in women of childbearing age in North America and industrialized nations [12–14]. Most cardiac patients being seen in relation to pregnancy, therefore, have CHD and we must understand the effects of pregnancy on these patients and the risks faced by the mother and her offspring to choose the best plan for ongoing management.

## Effects of pregnancy on the circulatory system

Important maternal cardiovascular adaptations start during the first trimester, peak in the late second and early third trimesters, and largely resolve by 6 weeks postpartum [12,15–17]. These adaptations are summarized in Table 1. Several recent reviews are available for more detailed descriptions of these hemodynamic changes [12,14–16].

The increases in stroke volume and heart rate [17] are preceded by a decrease in systemic vascular resistance evident early in the first trimester. This decrease in systemic vascular resistance is caused by the effects of pregnancy hormones and other vasoactive substances, including circulating prostaglandins [12,18–20]. The peripheral vasodilatation is accompanied by an increased glomerular filtration rate and may be the trigger for sodium and water retention [18,19], resulting in the increased circulating volume. There is

Dr. Kafka has been supported through the Detweiler Fellowship of the Royal College of Physicians and Surgeons of Canada and through a grant from the Department of Medicine at Queen's University, Canada.

* Corresponding author. Division of Cardiology, Queen's University Cardiovascular Laboratory, Kingston General Hospital, 76 Stewart Street, Kingston, ON, Canada K7L2V7.

E-mail address: kafkamd@usa.net (H. Kafka).

Table 1
Cardiovascular adaptations during pregnancy

| Parameter | Average change during pregnancy |
|---|---|
| Blood volume | ⇑ 35% |
| Cardiac output | ⇑ 40%–43% |
| Stroke volume | ⇑ 30% |
| Heart rate | ⇑ 15%–17% |
| Systemic vascular resistance | ⇓ 15%–21% |
| Mean arterial pressure | No significant change |
| Systolic blood pressure | ⇓ 3–5 mm Hg |
| Diastolic blood pressure | ⇓ 5–10 mm Hg |
| Central venous pressure | No significant change |
| Serum colloid osmotic pressure | ⇓ 14% |
| Hemoglobin | ⇓ 2.1 g/dL |
| $O_2$ consumption | ⇑ 30% |
| Right Ventricle (end diastole)[a] | ⇑ 18% |
| Right Atrium[a] | ⇑ 19% |
| Left Ventricle (end diastole)[a] | ⇑ 6% |
| Left Atrium[a] | ⇑ 12% |

[a] Echocardiographic dimensions.
*Adapted and modified from* Abbas AE, Lester SJ, Connolly H. Pregnancy and the cardiovascular system. Int J Card 2005;98:179–89.

pregnancy-associated enlargement of the cardiac chambers (Table 1), which is more apparent in the right-sided chambers [21]. The peripheral vasodilatation can be associated with postural symptoms, and caval pressure from the gravid uterus may exacerbate hypotension further [22].

Labor and delivery bring their own cardiovascular changes and challenges. The pain and anxiety during labor can increase heart rate and stroke volume. A further 300 to 500 mL of blood is transfused into the circulation with each uterine contraction and these factors combined can result in cardiac output increases of as much as 80% above prepregnancy levels [16]. Use of an epidural anesthetic can modulate these increases in cardiac output. About 500 mL of blood is lost during a normal vaginal delivery and a normal cesarean delivery is expected to result in the loss of 600 to 1000 mL. After delivery, there is relief of the caval compression and a further augmentation of maternal circulating volume by the return of blood from the placental sinusoids [12]. There has been some suggestion that this sudden augmentation of volume may lead to elevated levels of atrial natriuretic peptide and postpartum diuresis [23].

Changes in the structure of arteries and veins have been documented during pregnancy, and estrogen receptors have been found in human aortic tissue. A gradual dilatation of the aorta, renal, and placental vessels deals with the increased volume and cardiac output [24–26].

There is a significant increase in the procoagulant activity linked to elevations in factors V, VII, VIII, IX, X, XII, von Willebrand factor, and fibrinogen that peaks around term. These changes help to prevent hemorrhage during endovascular trophoblastic invasion and with hemostasis during delivery but they are associated with an increased incidence of thromboembolic complications [27]. It has been estimated that the risk for a thrombotic event is 6 times higher in pregnancy and 11 times higher in the puerperium [28].

Although the described changes are of benefit in the setting of a normal maternal circulation, these same changes can be challenging for the mother who has CHD and these challenges rise with the increasing complexity of the lesions. Patients who have shunts (ventricular septal defect [VSD], atrial septal defect [ASD]) and valvular regurgitation (pulmonary regurgitation, aortic regurgitation) generally tolerate this added volume load and increased cardiac output well. The presence of heart failure or symptoms before the pregnancy, however, can increase the risks even in this group. It is obvious that patients who have severe obstructive lesions (aortic stenosis, pulmonary stenosis) and those who have severe pulmonary hypertension cope poorly with the hemodynamic changes of pregnancy because of their limited ability to augment cardiac output. Those who have poor ventricular function may be expected to have similar difficulties [13,29]. One result of the plasma volume expansion is reduced serum colloid osmotic pressure and, in consequence, a lowered threshold for pulmonary edema [14].

The situation is further complicated for the patient who has cyanotic heart disease. These patients have chronic erythrocytosis and their own underlying hemostatic disorder which, coupled with the thrombophilic tendencies of pregnancy, could be expected to further increase the thromboembolic risks. Moreover, the drop in systemic vascular resistance may predispose to increased right-to-left shunting and, consequently, worsening maternal and fetal hypoxemia [9,12,15].

Marfan syndrome, bicuspid aortic valve [24], and coarctation [3] have all been associated with an increased risk for aortic dissection linked to their underlying aortopathy. This risk is further enhanced during pregnancy as a result of pregnancy-related tissue changes and the increased hemodynamic stresses on the aorta, being especially high in Marfan syndrome when the aortic root exceeds 4 cm [24]. Aortic root enlargement has been described in repaired tetralogy of Fallot [14,30] but the dissection risk in pregnant patients has not been reported.

In addition to the abnormal response of the patient who has CHD to the normal cardiovascular adaptations of pregnancy, there are the complications that can occur even in normal patients during pregnancy. Preeclampsia can seriously threaten a patient who has CHD (especially any form of pulmonary hypertension) because of the hypertension, renal dysfunction, and disseminated intravascular coagulation [31]. Urinary tract infections are common in pregnancy and the fever-induced tachycardia and vasodilation may be poorly tolerated. Arrhythmias during pregnancy [32–35] can occur in seemingly well individuals and may be related to the direct electrophysiologic effects of hormones, the changes in autonomic tone, and the physiologic cardiac dilatation [17,21,36]. Not surprisingly, they are more common during labor and delivery. Tachyarrhythmias may decompensate the patient who has an obstructive lesion or poor systemic ventricular function.

## Risks

Any discussion about pregnancy needs to start with an understanding and an assessment of the associated risks. These risks fall into four categories, each of which requires careful discussion: maternal risk during pregnancy, fetal risk, risk for recurrence of CHD in the offspring, and risk for early parental loss or disability. It must be emphasized, however, that accurate risk assessment may not be available for every type of adult CHD situation and that even the most quoted reports are based on relatively small numbers of patients. An in-depth review has recently tabulated the wide range of maternal and fetal risks [37].

### Maternal risk during pregnancy

Over the past 80 years there has been a significant decrease in the maternal mortality rate from 1 in 250 to 1 in 10,000 [31]. The reported maternal mortality rates in CHD vary from 1 in 1000 [31] to as high as 1 in 2 for patients who have Eisenmenger syndrome. Although congenital disease is the most common cardiac lesion during pregnancy in industrialized nations, fewer than one third of cardiac deaths during pregnancy in the United

Kingdom from 1987 to 2002 were attributable to CHD [38]. Myocardial infarction, aortic dissection, and cardiomyopathy each accounted for about 20% of the cardiac deaths. During 2000 to 2002, suicide was the leading cause of maternal death in the United Kingdom, followed by cardiac disease and thromboembolism [38].

In general, increasing maternal risk is associated with anatomic complexity, severity of obstructive lesions, poor function of the systemic ventricle, poor functional class, and the presence and degree of cyanosis [28]. The CARPREG group validated their prediction rule by following 599 pregnancies, of which 445 involved congenital heart defects, and identifying those who had primary cardiac events (pulmonary edema, stroke, tachyarrhythmia or bradyarrhythmia requiring treatment, cardiac arrest, or cardiac death). Thirteen percent of these patients suffered a primary cardiac event. This finding established four reliable predictors of these primary cardiac events:

- Prior cardiac event (CHF, transient ischemic attack, stroke) or symptomatic arrhythmias requiring treatment
- Baseline New York Heart Association (NYHA) greater than class II, or cyanosis
- Left heart obstruction (mitral valve area $< 2\,cm^2$, aortic valve area $< 1.5\,cm^2$, or peak left ventricular outflow gradient $> 30$ mm Hg by Doppler echocardiography)
- Reduced systemic ventricular function (ejection fraction $< 40\%$).

In the absence of any of these predictors, the risk for a primary cardiac event was 5%, rising to 27% in the presence of one predictor and to 75% when there were two or more predictors (there were no patients who had Eisenmenger syndrome in this study) [13]. A recent study of 90 pregnancies in women who had exclusively CHD has validated the CARPREG index score and has demonstrated that cardiac risk assessment could be improved further by adding decreased subpulmonary ventricular systolic function or severe pulmonary regurgitation to the CARPREG risk index [29]. In fact, mothers who had severe pulmonary regurgitation or reduced subpulmonary ventricular ejection fraction were 10 times more likely to have a cardiac complication. In addition to these predictors, a thorough knowledge of the patient's congenital heart lesion is necessary to deal with the specific risks of different types of lesions. These can be organized into low, moderate, and high risk and examples are presented in Tables 2, 3, and 4 [28].

Table 2
Lesions associated with low maternal risk

| Lesion | Exclude before pregnancy | Potential hazards | Recommended treatment during pregnancy and peripartum |
|--------|--------------------------|-------------------|-------------------------------------------------------|
| VSD | Pulmonary arterial hypertension | Arrhythmias<br>Endocarditis (unoperated or residual VSD) | Antibiotic prophylaxis for unoperated or residual VSD |
| ASD (unoperated) | Pulmonary arterial hypertension<br>Ventricular dysfunction | Arrhythmias<br>Thromboembolic events | Thromboprophylaxis if bed rest is required<br>Consider low-dose aspirin during pregnancy |
| Coarctation (repaired) | Recoarctation<br>Aneurysm formation at the site of repair (MRI)<br>Associated lesion, such as bicuspid aortic valve (+/− aortic stenosis or aortic regurgitation), ascending aortopathy<br>Systemic hypertension<br>Ventricular dysfunction | Preeclampsia<br>Aortic dissection<br>Congestive heart failure<br>Endarteritis | Beta blockers if necessary to control systemic blood pressure<br>Consider elective cesarean section before term in case of aortic aneurysm formation or uncontrollable systemic hypertension<br>Antibiotic prophylaxis |
| Tetralogy of Fallot (repaired) | Severe right ventricular outflow tract obstruction<br>Severe pulmonary regurgitation<br>Right ventricular dysfunction<br>DiGeorge syndrome (present in up to 15% of patients) | Arrhythmias<br>Right ventricular failure<br>Endocarditis | Consider preterm delivery in the rare case of right ventricular failure<br>Antibiotic prophylaxis |

*From* Uebing A, Steer PJ, Yentis SM, et al. Pregnancy and congenital heart disease. BMJ 2006;332:401–6.

To apply these prognostic indicators, one needs to have completed a thorough assessment of the patient, including history, physical examination, echocardiography, and relevant blood work, if indicated. In some patients it may be necessary to proceed to exercise testing, MRI, or cardiac catheterization to make as reliable an assessment as possible regarding prognosis and risk for the pregnancy.

*Fetal risk*

In a pregnancy complicated by preexisting heart disease, the fetus may be at greater risk for the usual pregnancy complications of prematurity and growth restriction but also may be exposed to the risks of lower maternal oxygen levels, drugs given to support the maternal cardiovascular state, and inheritance of a congenital cardiovascular condition. Prematurity carries with it the potential complications of respiratory distress syndrome, intracranial hemorrhage, and necrotizing enterocolitis. When prematurity is combined with growth restriction these problems are magnified several-fold, and inevitably these pregnancies are complicated by increased rates of stillbirth and neonatal death [39]. The same risk factors that predict maternal complications also can predict fetal and neonatal adverse effects, namely NYHA class greater than II, cyanosis, or important left heart obstruction [13,39]. The risk to the fetus is heightened further by smoking, maternal age (<20 or >35), and therapy with anticoagulants [13,29]. In general, fetal mortality reports have ranged from 6% to 24% [37] but can be as high as 50% in Eisenmenger syndrome [40]. For

Table 3
Lesions associated with moderate maternal risk

| Lesion | Exclude before pregnancy | Potential hazards | Recommended treatment during pregnancy and peripartum |
|---|---|---|---|
| Mitral stenosis | Severe stenosis Pulmonary venous hypertension | Atrial fibrillation Thromboembolic events Pulmonary edema | Beta blockers Low-dose aspirin Consider bed rest during the third trimester with additional thromboprophylaxis Antibiotic prophylaxis |
| Aortic stenosis | Severe stenosis (peak pressure gradient on Doppler > 80 mm Hg, ST segment depression, symptoms) Left ventricular dysfunction | Arrhythmias Angina Endocarditis Left ventricular failure | Bed rest during third trimester with thromboprophylaxis Consider balloon aortic valvotomy (for severe symptomatic valvar stenosis) or preterm cesarean section if cardiac decompensation ensues (cardiopulmonary bypass carries a 20% risk for fetal death) Antibiotic prophylaxis |
| Systemic right ventricle: TGA after atrial switch procedure; ccTGA | Ventricular dysfunction Severe systemic AV valve regurgitation Arrhythmias (brady- and tachyarrhythmias) Heart failure (NHYA > II) Obstruction of venous pathways after atrial switch as venous blood flow significantly increases during pregnancy | Right ventricular dysfunction (potentially persisting after pregnancy) Heart failure Arrhythmias Thromboembolic events Endocarditis | Regular monitoring of heart rhythm Restore sinus rhythm in case of atrial flutter (DC cardioversion usually effective and safe) Alter afterload reduction therapy (stop ACE inhibitors; consider beta blockers) Low-dose aspirin (81 mg) Antibiotic prophylaxis |
| Cyanotic lesions without pulmonary hypertension | Ventricular dysfunction | Hemorrhage (bleeding diathesis) Thromboembolic events Increased cyanosis Heart failure Endocarditis | Consider bed rest and oxygen supplementation to maintain oxygen saturation and promote oxygen tissue delivery (thromboprophylaxis with low molecular weight heparin) Antibiotic prophylaxis |
| Fontan-type circulation | Ventricular dysfunction Arrhythmias Heart failure (NYHA > II) | Heart failure Arrhythmias Thromboembolic complications Endocarditis | Consider anticoagulation with low molecular weight heparin and aspirin throughout pregnancy Maintain sufficient filling pressures and avoid dehydration during delivery Antibiotic prophylaxis |

*Abbreviations*: ACE, angiotensin converting enzyme; AV, atrioventricular, ccTGA, congenitally corrected TGA; TGA, transposition of the great arteries.
*From* Uebing A, Steer PJ, Yentis SM, et al. Pregnancy and congenital heart disease. BMJ 2006;332:401–6.

Table 4
Lesions associated with high maternal risk

| Lesion | Exclude before pregnancy | Potential hazards | Recommended treatment during pregnancy and peripartum |
|---|---|---|---|
| Marfan syndrome | Aortic root dilatation >4 cm | Type A dissection of the aorta | Beta blockers in all patients Elective cesarean section when aortic root >45 mm (~35 weeks of gestation) |
| Eisenmenger syndrome; other pulmonary arterial hypertension | Ventricular dysfunction Arrhythmias | 30%–50% risk for death related to pregnancy Arrhythmia Heart failure Endocarditis for Eisenmenger syndrome | Therapeutic termination should be offered If pregnancy continues close cardiovascular monitoring, early bed rest, pulmonary vasodilator therapy with supplemental oxygen should be considered Close monitoring necessary for 10 days postpartum |

*From* Uebing A, Steer PJ, Yentis SM, et al. Pregnancy and congenital heart disease. BMJ 2006;332:401–6.

the cyanotic patient, hemoglobin level and oxygen saturation are powerful predictors of fetal outcome. In women who have cyanotic congenital lesions, a hemoglobin of 16 or less was associated with a live birth rate of 71%, whereas the live birth rate fell to 8% when hemoglobin was 20 or higher. In a similar way, there was a 92% live birth rate for those who had oxygen saturation of 90 or higher but only 12% for those who had oxygen saturation of 85 or less [41].

Prematurity is associated not only with an increased risk for neonatal death but also with significant long-term morbidity [42,43], including cerebral palsy and bronchopulmonary dysplasia with its associated oxygen dependency for the surviving neonate. Maternal cyanosis, obstructive lesions, or poor ventricular function can result in the failure to meet the oxygen and nutrient demands of the fetus adequately, slowing fetal growth and sometimes requiring early delivery. Intrauterine growth restriction has been shown to have important long-term consequences ranging from neurodevelopment to vascular abnormality, diabetes, and dyslipidemia [44]. By detecting growth restriction as early as possible, we can initiate therapy to improve both the maternal situation and the fetus. If that is not possible, or is unsuccessful, steps need to be taken to plan the optimal delivery time, including the use of

steroids to mature fetal lungs if the delivery is necessary before 34 weeks. Ultrasound assessments to monitor fetal growth should be done every 2 to 4 weeks depending on the clinical situation [31].

*Risk for recurrence of congenital heart disease in the offspring*

The overall risk for any child being born with CHD is estimated at 0.8%, whereas the risk for a structural cardiac lesion in the offspring of a parent who has CHD ranges from 2% to 50% (Table 5) with a wide range of these recurrence risks reported in several studies [28,37,45–49]. The recurrence risk seems to depend on the parent's specific cardiac defect and on which parent is affected. There is a general impression that the risk for recurrence may be higher if the mother is the affected parent [37,46] but this does not hold true for all defects or all reports. Of course, the recurrence rate in autosomal dominant lesions such as Holt-Oram, or Marfan syndrome is 50%. Special attention needs to be paid to the clinical syndromes that are part of the wide spectrum of 22q11 deletions. Once believed to be a rare cause of DiGeorge syndrome, it is now apparent that 22q11 deletions are far more common [48,50]. They may be detected in up to 50% of children born with interrupted arch or persistent truncus

Table 5
Recurrence risk for congenital heart disease

| CHD defect | Risk for Recurrence (%) | |
| --- | --- | --- |
| | Mother affected | Father affected |
| Atrioventricular septal defect | 7.9–13.9 | 4.3–7.7 |
| Aortic stenosis | 8.0–13.9 | 3.8 |
| Coarctation | 4.1–6.3 | 3.0–6.0 |
| Atrial septal defect | 4.6–11 | 1.5–3.6 |
| Ventricular septal defect | 6.0–15.6 | 3.0–3.6 |
| Pulmonary stenosis | 5.3–6.5 | 2.0–3.5 |
| Persistent ductus arteriosus | 4.1 | 2.0–2.5 |
| Tetralogy of Fallot[a] | 2.0–4.5 | 1.6 |
| Marfan syndrome | 50 | 50 |
| 22q11 deletion syndromes | 50 | 50 |

[a] Assuming that the parent does not have 22q11 deletion.

*Data from* Refs. [28,37,45–49].

arteriosus and 10% to 15% of children who have tetralogy of Fallot or pulmonary atresia. Associated defects, such as facial dysmorphism, nasal speech, learning difficulties, cleft palate, hearing impairment, psychiatric illness, or talipes equinovarus, are clues to possible 22q11 deletions, but there are individuals with an isolated cardiac or vascular defect who have a 22q11 deletion and run a 50% risk for passing that deletion to an offspring [48,50]. The contribution of a clinical geneticist in these complex cases is invaluable.

Because of the greater risk for CHD in the offspring of a parent who has congenital heart disease, consideration should be given to offering ultrasound scans to screen for congenital lesions [28,31]. A normal fetal nuchal translucency measurement at 12 to 13 weeks has a negative predictive value of 99.9% for fetal heart disease and can be used to reassure a parent who has congenital heart disease. For those who have a strong family history of congenital heart disease, a specialist fetal echocardiogram should be performed at 14 to 16 weeks. This scan can detect moderate to severe lesions but cannot rule out all forms of CHD because the fetal heart is so small at this stage. This test needs to be followed up with a further echocardiographic scan at 18 to 22 weeks [31,51].

*Risk for early parental loss or disability*

Becoming a parent carries a serious responsibility to care for the child, including nurturing,

loving, and providing financially for the child. These matters should be considered by a potential parent who has congenital heart disease. Adults who have CHD may have difficulty obtaining health insurance [6,8]. Some patients have an increased risk for premature death and disability or may have to face the possibility of repeated major surgery [3,5]. These issues must be discussed despite their difficulty. The matter of mortality and the fact that the patient has not been "cured" may come up for the first time in these discussions. Although the physician wants to be as frank as possible, the data about patient prognosis is constantly changing with improvements and innovations in cardiac care and all involved must understand that discussions about prognosis can only involve generalizations. The patient may benefit from the skill and counseling of a psychologist or psychiatrist or advanced practice nurse with experience in such situations.

## Care of the patient (Appendix 1)

*Prepregnancy care and counseling*

Individuals who have CHD need to be counseled about reproductive issues as they reach adolescence. This need cannot be overemphasized because up to 80% of pregnancies in teenagers are unplanned [52]. We know that an unplanned pregnancy can be a life-altering event for any teenager, but it can be life-threatening for those who have CHD. Counseling and teaching thus should take place long before the patient reaches the adult congenital heart clinic [6,53] and the pediatric cardiologist needs to ensure that such counseling has occurred. It has been reported that some parents of adolescent patients tend to regard their maturing offspring as asexual [6] and avoid questions about sexuality or reproduction. As a consequence, these adolescents harbor misconceptions and fears about their sexual function and ability to conceive, and the dangers associated with pregnancy. They have reported fears about death during sexual activity and fears about transmitting their cardiac defect to offspring [6]. Because some CHD may be accompanied by intellectual impairment, these counseling sessions may be challenging and require judgment and sensitivity in addressing all the relevant issues. Frank discussions about sexual activity and reproductive issues may be hampered by the presence of a parent or guardian. This same difficulty also can be present in the adult clinic because these young women and men have been patients since birth and often continue to be accompanied by their parents during clinic visits. Patients, both adults and adolescents, should be given the opportunity to meet with their caregivers for at least part of their visits without their parents so that they can ask questions, answer questions, and receive information not only about sexual functioning but also about their heart condition and prognosis.

When the patient arrives in the adult clinic, one cannot assume that she (or he) has a full understanding of the reproductive issues. The patient may be reluctant to receive counseling because there are no plans to start a family in the near future. Counseling and education should be offered to everyone so that patients, male and female, understand the general risks inherent for themselves and their offspring and the more specific risks concerning their particular congenital defect and repair. There needs to be careful and sensitive discussion about the residual defects or expected deterioration that would increase pregnancy risks or significantly limit life expectancy. This discussion is done not to impose the physician's opinions onto the patient but to provide the information and the teaching necessary to allow the patient to make the most appropriate decision about future parenthood and contraception. These discussions should not be limited to female patients because the issues of risk for recurrence and risk for premature parental disability or loss apply to fathers also.

To provide the best information about risks to the patient, it is necessary to have a thorough understanding of the congenital defect and the outcomes of the previous surgical and catheter interventions in that patient. This testing may be more comprehensive than is routine to give a clear and informed picture. Furthermore, to decrease risk during pregnancy, one may even consider surgical or catheter interventions that might otherwise have been postponed to a later date. Such procedures can be justified clearly in the preparations for a planned pregnancy because catheter and surgical interventions during pregnancy carry their own special risks [28,54] and certain residual defects markedly increase maternal and fetal risks.

## Contraception

Even in patients who do not have CHD any discussion about contraception must deal with the issues of compliance, reliability, and safety. These discussions need to involve an obstetrician who is familiar with the special challenges of contraception in patients who have CHD because there is no ideal contraceptive method. The consequences of an unplanned pregnancy in this group of patients can be grave, and despite recommendations, contraceptive teaching is not always successful, with one study reporting that 6 of 35 women who had CHD had an unplanned pregnancy [55]. A complete recent review of contraception for patients who have CHD is available [31].

Because of their unacceptable failure rates, natural methods of birth control cannot be recommended for patients in the high and moderate maternal risk groups (see Tables 3 and 4) Barrier methods (condom and diaphragm) have failure rates of 2% to 50% depending on the compliance with their use. Spermicidal jelly or cream is recommended to be used in conjunction with the condom or diaphragm. These barrier methods may end up being the best choice for women who face unacceptably high risks with the other techniques. In the case of failure of contraception in the high maternal risk group, early termination of pregnancy should be given due consideration.

The oral contraceptive pill remains a popular technique among young women. There are two categories of oral contraceptive: the combined pill with estrogen and progestogen, and the low-dose pill (or mini-pill) that contains a very low dose of progestogen. The combined pill is significantly more effective, with a failure rate of less than 1 per 1000 women per year. Because it is associated with a fourfold increased risk for thrombosis [31], however, it cannot be recommended for the woman who already has a defect that predisposes to thrombosis (cyanosis, atrial arrhythmias, valvular prostheses, Fontan-type circulations). Conversely, it may be a good choice for the lower-risk patient because of its effectiveness. In comparison, the low-dose progestogen pill does not predispose to thrombosis but is not as effective, with a failure rate of 1 in 200 per year. Furthermore, its effectiveness depends on close compliance to a rigid daily regimen and therefore it is not a good choice for most adolescents [52]. In those cases, an alternative hormonal approach may involve the use of an injectable progestogen.

Intrauterine devices generally had not been recommended for these patients because of their previous association with menorrhagia, increased risk for pelvic infections, and bacteremias [6,16]. A newer generation of a progestogen-impregnated device actually reduces menstrual bleeding (amenorrhea is common) and has a low risk for pelvic infection or ectopic pregnancy [28]. The progestogen coating carries no increased risk for thromboembolism and these coils can be left in place for five years, thus eliminating any compliance issues [31]. The actual process of coil insertion, regardless of type, may carry a risk for endocarditis and requires antibiotic prophylaxis against genitourinary organisms. Occasionally the insertion procedure may be complicated by a vasovagal reaction that could be poorly tolerated by an individual who has unstable hemodynamics [16]. It has been recommended that coil insertions for such women be done in the operating room with the anesthesia staff present [31].

Sterilization can be considered for the patient who has decided to avoid pregnancy permanently or who has decided not to have any more children. The procedure is done by laparoscopy and carries an anesthetic and surgical risk that can be substantial for the patient who has complex anatomy or Eisenmenger syndrome. The risk for pregnancy after sterilization has been considered to be between 0.2% and 1% per year [31]. Occasionally, a young patient who has a fear of pregnancy may request sterilization, often with urging from her family. Such requests should be met with careful explanation and exploration of options before proceeding [6].

Vasectomy is a low-risk option for the male patient who has decided not to have offspring and it can be considered for the male partner of a woman who has congenital heart disease. The couple may decide against vasectomy if the woman's life expectancy is likely to be shorter and the man may wish to have children with a future partner.

*Termination*

When contraception fails, a decision needs to be made quickly about whether to carry on with the pregnancy or to proceed to termination because the risks of termination, although small, do increase with advancing gestational age. In general, one can state that termination of pregnancy is about half as dangerous as continuation with the pregnancy [31]. Dilation and suction curettage under local anesthetic carries a low complication rate as a first-trimester procedure, but for those at moderate and high risk it should be performed in a hospital operating room rather than in an outpatient setting [52]. Medical abortion with oral antiprogesterones

and vaginally administered prostaglandins is effective in the first 7 weeks but again must be performed in hospital because there are several unpredictable effects, such as systemic vasodilatation and heavy bleeding, that may contribute to hypotension and destabilize the patient. Certainly medical abortion is not to be considered for patients who have Eisenmenger syndrome (or other types of pulmonary hypertension) or for those who have cyanosis.

The decision to terminate may be made for personal or medical reasons. An unplanned pregnancy in a moderate- (see Table 3) or high-risk patient (see Table 4) could be considered a medical indication for termination. If the patient wishes to continue with the pregnancy, she should be referred to a high-risk multidisciplinary tertiary care center clinic.

*Prenatal care*

With thoughtful investigation and assessment, a plan for prenatal care should be established before the patient becomes pregnant. If that has not occurred, it is important to generate such a plan as soon as possible in the pregnancy. In this way, the criteria previously described can be used to rate the risk of the patient. Low-risk patients (see Table 2) can receive their prenatal care from their usual specialists, with ongoing advice available from the high-risk pregnancy team at the tertiary center. Patients whose risk profile is moderate and high (see Tables 3 and 4) should be referred to the team with the plan that labor and delivery will occur at that tertiary center.

Like other prenatal clinic visits, these focus on monitoring fetal growth and development but also include a CHD screening ultrasound and a close assessment of the mother's cardiovascular status at each visit, looking for symptoms and signs of heart failure, arrhythmia, or endocarditis. Such complications may be precipitated by problems, such as anemia or urinary tract infection, which, although minor in a healthy woman, are of greater significance in a woman who has preexisting heart disease. Preeclampsia can be particularly disastrous in the setting of complex congenital defects and especially so for patients who have Eisenmenger syndrome and it must be specifically sought out. A planned program for prenatal visits has been described by Steer [31] and its intensity depends on the assessed maternal risk. For moderate- to high-risk patients, frequent visits are recommended—every 2 weeks until 24 weeks and then weekly thereafter—along with special antenatal records designed for the care of pregnant women who have heart disease (see Fig. 1). Planned echocardiography is necessary for patients at risk for aortic root dilatation and should be used liberally for any patient who has a new murmur or suspicion of clinical deterioration. Radiographs should be avoided if at all possible, and all the usual precautions need to be taken if radiologic examination is necessary [56]. Cardiovascular MRI generally is accepted to be safe in the setting of pregnancy [57]. There is no human evidence to suggest risk to the fetus during the first trimester but until the absolute safety of MRI

during the susceptible period can be established, it is best to avoid scans in the first trimester except situations in which the benefits outweigh the potential risks [57].

Some patients require hospitalization during the third trimester for treatment of complications, for bed rest or closer monitoring, and for oxygen therapy in cyanotic patients [28]. Because of the thrombophilia of pregnancy, it is important that these pregnant patients on bed rest receive low molecular weight heparin (LMWH) and antithromboembolism stockings.

There is no clear consensus with regard to endocarditis prophylaxis at the time of delivery.

## Antenatal records for women with cardiac disease

Name:                              Cardiac lesion
S/B cardiologist                   S/B Anaesthetist
Fetal cardiac scan                 Fetal anomaly scan

EDD:                               Delivery plan:

| Date |  |  |  |  |  |  |
|---|---|---|---|---|---|---|
| Gestation |  |  |  |  |  |  |
| SOB |  |  |  |  |  |  |
| Palpitations |  |  |  |  |  |  |
| Other symptoms |  |  |  |  |  |  |
| BP |  |  |  |  |  |  |
| Pulse rate |  |  |  |  |  |  |
| Pulse rhythm |  |  |  |  |  |  |
| Murmur |  |  |  |  |  |  |
| Lung bases |  |  |  |  |  |  |
| Oedema |  |  |  |  |  |  |
| SFH |  |  |  |  |  |  |
| Presentation |  |  |  |  |  |  |
| 5ths palp |  |  |  |  |  |  |
| FH |  |  |  |  |  |  |
| Urine |  |  |  |  |  |  |
| Next appt |  |  |  |  |  |  |
| Signature |  |  |  |  |  |  |

Fig. 1. Example of antenatal record for women who has cardiac disease. This record facilitates ongoing documentation of findings and progress during the antenatal visits. The observations at each visit are cardiac and obstetric, designed to detect any maternal or fetal problems at an early stage. The cardiac diagnosis (lesion) needs to be as specific as possible. The form provides space for notes about fetal cardiac and anomaly ultrasound examinations. The plan for delivery (elective cesarean section or trial of labor) should be noted. 5ths palp, amount of fetal head palpable; appt, appointment; BP, blood pressure; EDD, estimated date of delivery; FH, fetal heart; S/B, seen by; SFH, symphysis/fundal height; SOB, short of breath. (Courtesy of Philip Steer and the High Risk Obstetric Team, Chelsea and Westminster Hospital, London UK.)

The current American Heart Association guidelines do not call for routine prophylaxis for uncomplicated delivery. Nevertheless, because of the devastating consequences of endocarditis in this setting, some centers routinely give IV antibiotics to patients who have high-risk lesions [16], whereas others use prophylaxis selectively for the patient who has any form of instrumented vaginal delivery or cesarean section [31].

Thromboembolism is six times more common during pregnancy [28], even for women who do not have congenital heart disease. There is an even greater risk for the cyanotic patient and the patient who has a Fontan circulation. The patient who has a left-to-right shunt faces a risk for paradoxic embolism even in the nonpregnant state and that risk is probably enhanced during pregnancy. Low-dose aspirin [22,58] can be used safely for these patients until the 36th week of pregnancy. A major challenge is the management of chronic anticoagulation throughout pregnancy, especially in the patient who has a prosthetic valve [9,59,60]. Warfarin crosses the placenta, has teratogenic effects early in pregnancy, and poses increased risks of fetal hemorrhage during pregnancy, whereas heparin does not cross the placenta and is safer for the fetus but is associated with more maternal thromboembolism [59,60]. The American College of Chest Physicians (ACCP) Conference on Antithrombotic Therapy has recommended one of three regimens, namely, using unfractionated heparin (UFH), LMWH, or a combination of warfarin and heparin (Box 1) for pregnant patients. There is a fourth option of continuing warfarin throughout pregnancy until the 36th week in the high-risk valve patient and then using heparin until delivery [28], but this approach is rarely used in North America because of concerns about warfarin embryopathy and fetal hemorrhage [60]. For patients at high risk because of prosthetic heart valves, one may consider the addition of low-dose aspirin, despite the fact that there are no data concerning this combined use in pregnancy [60].

Atrial arrhythmias occur commonly during pregnancy and may not be well tolerated if associated with decreases in cardiac output [37]. Antiarrhythmic drugs should be avoided if at all possible; however, adenosine, digoxin, procainamide, flecainide, quinidine, and calcium channel blockers generally are accepted as safe [28,58]. There had been concerns about the use of beta blockers because of a past association with intrauterine growth restriction. Although this risk is now considered small, close monitoring for

---

**Box 1. Recommended regimens for the management of anticoagulation through pregnancy from the Seventh ACCP Conference on Antithrombotic Therapy (2004)**

Each of these is a Grade 1C recommendation; that is, the risk-to-benefit ratio is clearly favorable but it is based largely on observational studies and should be considered to be an intermediate-strength recommendation that may change when stronger evidence is available.

OR

Adjusted-dose, twice-daily LMWH throughout pregnancy in doses adjusted either to keep a 4-hour postinjection anti-Xa heparin level at approximately 1.0 to 1.2 U/mL (preferable) or according to weight

OR

Aggressive adjusted-dose UFH throughout pregnancy (ie, administered SC every 12 hours in doses adjusted to keep the mid-interval activated partial thromboplastin time at least twice control or to attain an anti-Xa heparin level of 0.35 to 0.70 U/mL)

OR

UFH or LMWH (as above) until the 13th week, change to warfarin until the middle of the third trimester, and then restart UFH or LMWH.

---

*Abbreviations:* LMWH, low molecular weight heparin; SC, subcutaneously; UFH, unfractionated heparin. *From* Bates SM, Greer IA, Hirsh J, et al. Use of antithrombotic agents during pregnancy. Chest 2004;126:627S–44S.

---

growth restriction is recommended. Lidocaine or sotalol can be used for ventricular tachycardia but amiodarone should be avoided if at all possible and used only under special circumstances [12,37,58,61]. Direct current (DC) cardioversion is considered safe in the pregnant patient [9,15].

It is common for pregnant women who do not have heart disease to complain of fatigue, dyspnea, or pedal edema and it may be challenging to distinguish the signs and symptoms of a normal pregnancy from those of early heart failure [62]. Furthermore, even patients who had few symptoms before pregnancy can develop heart failure during the pregnancy. Pulmonary edema occurred in 42 of 599 pregnancies and 34 of these women had been in class I or II before the pregnancy [13]. Heart failure is associated with restricted fetal growth and prematurity and may require admission for optimization of medical treatment. Diuretics are relatively safe in pregnancy but angiotensin-converting enzyme inhibitors and angiotensin-receptor blockers are contraindicated [28,37,58]. Nitrates are safe and can be used with hydralazine for combined preload and afterload reduction in the pregnant patient [58,63,64]. Spironolactone is not recommended because of a potential to feminize the male fetus. Amiloride has been considered generally safe in pregnancy [28,58] but there have been reports of teratogenesis in rats [65]. Amiloride should be used only if potassium supplementation has not been effective.

There are patients who continue to deteriorate clinically despite optimal medical therapy. Depending on the stage of pregnancy, termination or early delivery may be considered. If termination or delivery are not options, then careful assessment needs to be performed to decide whether the patient may benefit from a surgical or catheter intervention. If surgery is considered, it is best to avoid cardiopulmonary bypass because of the significant associated fetal mortality. If cardiopulmonary bypass is necessary, the use of high flow/high pressure cardiopulmonary bypass and the avoidance of hypothermia are recommended. Catheter interventions may carry increased long-term radiation-associated risks to the child but have a low fetal mortality rate [54]. The most common interventions during pregnancy in patients who have CHD involve pulmonary or aortic valve stenosis. Fortunately such interventions rarely are required.

*Labor and delivery*

Because pregnant women can present at any time, day or night, with labor or urgent complications, there is a need for constant availability of staff and facilities. This availability is even more necessary for the medium- to high-risk CHD

patient. Any tertiary care center that is providing a high-risk joint cardiac obstetric service must be capable of providing full access to the proper facilities and the specialized labor and delivery team at all hours. This team would include the obstetrician, the anesthetist, the neonatologist, the cardiologist, and the intensivist, all of whom should be experienced in the management of the pregnant patient who has CHD.

Labor and delivery plans are made during the course of the clinic visits in consultation with the patient. There must be clear documentation of the plan with copies available to the team at all times, and to her local hospital if she lives some distance away. It is advisable to provide copies of the notes and delivery plans (Fig. 2) to the patient so that they are immediately available on her arrival. The process of planning and the issues surrounding labor and delivery have been described thoroughly in a recent review [31].

Previously, elective cesarean section under general anesthesia had been the chosen mode of delivery for many women who had congenital heart disease, in the belief that this would provide the most controlled environment for the delivery with the planned presence of the experienced team members and would avoid the stresses associated with pushing during the second stage of labor. Elective cesarean section, however, increases the risk for hemorrhage, thrombosis, and infection [31], and carries about 1.2 to 1.4 times the risk of a vaginal delivery. The stresses of labor can now be managed with the use of low-dose slow incremental epidural anesthesia, and with the availability of the high-risk team at all times there are no real advantages to elective cesarean section in these patients, except for obstetric indications.

Spontaneous labor is preferred to induced labor and it may be advisable to admit some patients who live a distance away to the tertiary center to await spontaneous delivery. Occasionally, it may be necessary to induce labor for obstetric reasons or in the face of cardiovascular decompensation [28]. With effective epidural anesthesia, uterine contractions usually have no evident adverse hemodynamic effects. The second stage of labor requires pushing and can have detrimental effects if prolonged. Part of the delivery plan, therefore, should establish how long the patient can push without significant hemodynamic compromise (see Fig. 2). Once that limit has been reached, delivery can be assisted by forceps or ventouse (vacuum) extraction [31]. After delivery, relief of caval obstruction increases venous

## Joint Cardiac Obstetric Service (JCOS) management plan for delivery

Cardiac diagnosis.........................................................................................

*Please circle agreed plan and tick box when actioned:*

If admitted to labour ward, Please inform:

Obstetrician on call          Consultant/registrar

Anaesthetist on call          Consultant/registrar

Cardiac team                  Y/N

Antenatal admission:          From ............ weeks

Mode of delivery: Elective lower caesarean section/trial of vaginal delivery

CAESAREAN SECTION:

        **Anaesthetic technique**: epidural/spinal/general/other

        **Maternal monitoring**: ECG/SaO₂/non-invasive BP/invasive BP/CVP

        **3rd stage**:       Prophylactic compression suture/Syntocinon 5 U over 10–20 min

                       /Syntocinon – low-dose infusion (8–12 mU/min)

Vaginal delivery 1st stage

        HDU chart/TEDS in labour/medication to be continued   ............

        **Prophylactic antibiotics**: Elective/if operative delivery

        Epidural for analgesia: none/when requested/as soon as in established labour

        Comments re anaesthetic  ..............................................................

        Maternal monitoring: ECG/SaO₂/non-invasive BP/invasive BP/CVP

Vaginal delivery 2nd stage

        Normal second stage/short second stage (then assist if not delivered within

        maximum min pushing)/elective assisted delivery only

Vaginal delivery 3rd stage

        Normal active management (oxytocin and CCT)/Syntocinon infusion 8–12 mU/min

        Continue Syntocinon infusion ...... h

Post delivery

        High Dependency Unit (min stay ......... h)/LMW heparin (duration ......)

        Other drugs postpartum .........

*Please inform the consultant obstetrician on call if there is departure from planned management or if new clinical situations develop.*

Fig. 2. Example of a delivery management plan for patients who have cardiac disease. The cardiac diagnosis needs to be as specific as possible. The form allows the physician to choose whether the cardiac team needs to be contacted immediately on admission and whether the patient will be admitted electively at a certain gestational age (number of weeks). A decision will have been made whether to proceed with elective cesarean section or to attempt a trial of vaginal delivery. For each situation there are several choices regarding anesthetic and monitoring. For vaginal delivery, a decision is made whether to allow any pushing or to provide a maximum time for pushing (minutes), after which assisted delivery is undertaken. Decisions about prophylactic antibiotics and which medications are to be continued are indicated on the form. Any postdelivery medication plans should be documented also. Plans for stay in the high-dependency unit (step-down unit) or intensive care unit will also be noted. BP, blood pressure; CCT, controlled cord traction; CVP, central venous pressure; EKG, electrocardiogram; HDU, high-dependency unit; LMW, low molecular weight heparin; SaO₂, oxygen saturations; TEDS, thromboembolic deterrent stockings. (Courtesy of Philip Steer and the High Risk Obstetric Team, Chelsea and Westminster Hospital, London UK.)

return and this is augmented by the transfusion of blood previously in the maternal placental bed. This return may overwhelm the patient's ability to cope with the extra volume load. Conversely, failure of uterine retraction may lead to uterine hemorrhage and a loss of volume. Oxytocic drugs can have marked hemodynamic effects and should be given cautiously at the lowest effective dosage, with close attention to the uterine response to avoid excessive blood loss.

A key to successful labor and delivery is the ongoing assessment of the fetal status and the mother's hemodynamic situation. Continuous fetal monitoring is necessary in these cases. Maternal monitoring includes continuous electro-cardiogram and pulse oximetry and measurement of blood pressure. Intra-arterial monitoring has the advantage of communicating rapid blood pressure changes [28,31] and is recommended in patients who have aortopathy (eg, Marfan, coarctation). A central venous line can be of value in the high-risk or decompensating patient but must be placed by an experienced operator with knowledge of the patient's complex anatomy. An in-line filter (air filter or bubble trap) for the intravenous line is recommended for any patient who has right-to-left shunting or a significant potential for right-to-left shunting.

Thrombotic risk is enhanced during the puerperium with most thromboembolic deaths occurring postpartum [38]. Prophylactic LMWH has been recommended for all patients in the moderate- and high-risk groups, selected patients in the lower-risk group, and all those having cesarean section [28,38]. Anticoagulation with heparin can be restarted safely within 6 to 12 hours after delivery and the mother can safely breastfeed. Warfarin usually is resumed in 48 hours but may need to be delayed in individuals at increased risk for postpartum hemorrhage. Although digoxin and flecainide do not enter breast milk in any significant amounts, beta blockers have been reported occasionally to cause bradycardia in the breastfed infant and should be used with careful monitoring of the infant [31,58,61].

There may be patient decompensation during any of these stages, including the puerperium, and careful maternal monitoring must continue throughout. In the event of clinical deterioration, there must be rapid access to the cardiologist and to an intensivist who understands the patient's complex underlying cardiac physiology. Ideally the intensivist would have been informed of the patient's admission to the labor room and would have had an opportunity to review the patient, the notes, and the plan of therapy.

## Summary

There can be significant risks for mother and offspring in the setting of parental congenital heart disease. The key to a happy outcome is early assessment and counseling and advanced planning through specialized centers and teams. A well-structured team should be able not only to direct the management of the pregnancy but also to provide guidance to the patient about issues relating to prognosis, sexual activity, contraception, genetic risks, and parental responsibility.

## Acknowledgments

The authors thank Dr. Alan Magee for his expert review of the manuscript and advice on the pediatric challenges in these patients and Professor Philip Steer and the High Risk Obstetric Team at the Chelsea and Westminster Hospital for permission to reproduce their forms.

## Appendix 1

*Organization of a multidisciplinary team for pregnancy and reproductive issues in the patient who has congenital heart disease*

### The team approach

The preceding sections have outlined the issues and management challenges in providing the best care for the CHD patient during her or his reproductive years. Neither the cardiologist nor the obstetrician alone has the training, experience, or expertise to deal with all the necessary aspects involved in the reproductive issues for these patients. A collaborative team approach is required and the members of the team change as the needs of the patient change. Such teams can be referred to as high-risk pregnancy teams but that term can be misleading and it may result in some patients not being referred because they are not pregnant, are not actively planning pregnancy, or are men. Any suggested alternative name (multi-disciplinary pregnancy or reproductive services clinic) tends to be just as awkward, however, and no less intimidating to the patient. The name of the clinic matters less than its composition and the training and expertise of its members. It may seem inappropriate to include a pediatric clinic in a discussion of the management of adult patients who have congenital heart disease, but the issues of reproductive health and pregnancy can be considered adult issues, regardless of whether they are addressed at the age of 14 or 18.

*Team 1: Pediatric reproductive issues team*

The patient who has CHD enters the reproductive period of her (or his) life long before transfer to the adult clinic. This means that the first assessment of, and discussion about, reproductive issues should take place in a pediatric setting [6]. The pediatric cardiologist has had years of ongoing cardiac assessment of this patient and usually has already discussed adolescent issues, such as body piercing and alcohol and tobacco use. The pediatric cardiologist is therefore in the best situation to discuss the issues of diagnosis and prognosis with the patient, and to ensure that the patient has had the opportunity to ask questions. The patient may feel more comfortable speaking with the advanced practice nurse assigned to the clinic or may benefit from meeting with a psychologist or psychiatrist to help deal with some of the difficult issues that may arise around prognosis. Female patients should be seen by an obstetrician (or by the family physician, pediatrician, or counselor) for an assessment and counseling about sexual activity and contraception. This topic may be awkward to broach with the patient and the family. In this type of situation, it may be best to inform the family and the patient that in the early teen years it is important to deal with issues of reproductive and gynecologic health for all patients, not just those who have increased cardiac risk. In this way, the referral is merely part of the usual care plan for all patients. The referral could be to the obstetrician who is already involved with the adult pregnancy clinic because he or she can discuss confidently the risks of future pregnancies based on the assessment and on the information from the pediatric cardiologist. Male patients, especially those who have heritable disorders, also would benefit from counseling about sexual activity and contraception. Depending on the nature of the congenital heart lesion and the patient's maturity and interest, he or she could be referred for an assessment and counseling by a clinical geneticist.

*Team 2: Adult reproductive issues team*

Once the patient has been referred to an adult cardiologist, no assumption should be made that any of the assessments or counseling recommended above has taken place [53]. It is necessary to determine what the patient knows, and, if the patient is agreeable, to arrange a referral to the adult reproductive issues team. This team should consist of a cardiologist with training and expertise in adult CHD and in the management of the pregnant patient, and an obstetrician with special interest and experience in the care of pregnant patients who have congenital heart disease. Ideally, the patient would have already seen the obstetrician for assessment but it has been reported that many women, even sexually active women, are not referred until their late 20s, 30s, or even after they become pregnant [6]. These two specialists make up the core of the team and can be supplemented when necessary with a clinical geneticist having experience in cardiovascular genetics and counseling, and a psychologist or psychiatrist to help the patient deal with some of the difficult aspects of his or her current clinical situation and prognosis. In addition, the advanced practice nurse assigned to the clinic can be a source of comfort and counseling for the patient. The cardiologist's assessment is based on information from the pediatric cardiologist and the referring cardiologist and is supplemented by a current examination and further investigation, if necessary. In this way, a risk profile can be established and decisions made about the risks of future pregnancy and the most appropriate form of contraception. Infertility issues also can be discussed and options presented. After the initial assessment and counseling are complete, the patient may return to her own clinic, to be referred back whenever necessary.

*Team 3: High-risk pregnancy team*

Once the patient is pregnant, she needs a referral to the high-risk pregnancy team. Ideally, she would have been assessed by Team 2 and would already have a well-documented risk profile. If not, the first step is to determine her risk status by whatever investigations can be carried out safely in her current stage of pregnancy. The second step is to determine if there are any medical reasons not to proceed with the pregnancy and to counsel the patient regarding that (keeping in mind that it is her decision whether to continue with the pregnancy), and the third step is to draw up the program for prenatal care. In addition to the cardiologist and the obstetrician, the anesthetist is an important member of this team and will want to assess the risks for epidural and for general anesthesia and explain all possible procedures and risks to the patient. Documentation of the prenatal plan and the plan for labor and delivery is crucial and it is essential that there is open access to this plan at all times so that it is available whenever the patient presents, or to advise another center should she present there.

*Team 4: High-risk labor and delivery team*

In addition to the cardiologist, obstetrician, and anesthetist, the team must include a neonatologist and an intensivist. Access to a pediatric cardiologist is advisable, especially if a screening ultrasound has revealed a cardiac defect. In the case of an autosomal dominant lesion in the parent, a referral for a pediatric cardiology assessment is prudent, even in the absence of a fetal cardiac defect. The intensivist should be alerted early in the course of labor and should have an understanding of the patient's cardiac defect and how her altered physiology and hemodynamics may complicate any intensive care unit stay. Because the patient may present at any time with labor or complications, team members must be available at all times with complete access to the notes and plans that have been so carefully laid out in the clinic. The goal is to have an uneventful delivery with most contingencies planned for, in the presence of experienced specialists whose expertise allows them to react quickly in the case of complications [9,31].

*Frequently asked questions*

*It is difficult to arrange to have all these specialists in one clinic at any time. Do they all have to see the patient at the same time?*

Ideally, the patient should see all the team members at her first assessment so that she gets a real understanding of their roles and interactions and the team members can freely discuss the situation among themselves and with the patient. It is acceptable to have the team members see the patient in separate locations and at separate times but the need to have open communication and full access to notes and plans cannot be overemphasized. Subsequent visits (eg, prenatal monitoring) do not need to involve all team members unless there have been concerns.

*Which patient needs to be referred to these clinics?*

If the patient's cardiologist believes that she is in the low-risk group (see Table 2), she does not necessarily need to be referred to the clinic. It may be prudent, however, to refer all patients for an initial assessment and risk profile by the experienced specialists in the clinic. They then can put together a plan for the patient to take back with her.

Furthermore, they will be available for advice and consultation at a distance should there be any problems. For patients in the moderate- and high-risk group, arrangements will be made for prenatal visits and delivery at the clinic center.

*The high-risk clinic is a long distance away from the patient's home. Would it not be more convenient for the patient to be seen and delivered locally?*

It would be more convenient but in the case of moderate- and high-risk patients it cannot be recommended. The benefits to mother and child of the facilities and staff at the tertiary center's high-risk clinic outweigh any inconvenience because of distance. Lack of insurance and financial support can be a problem, especially in the United States, and pose a dilemma to the patient and her family. In those cases, close liaison with the local specialists on a regular basis may replace the need for some of the prenatal visits but one cannot overemphasize the need to be delivered at the high-risk center.

*What if the patient goes into premature labor?*

There should already be a plan for dealing with the situation of premature labor for any patient who lives some distance away. Depending on the progress of labor and the patient's cardiac situation, urgent transfer may be possible, but early communication with the high-risk clinic is important. The patient should have copies of her notes and plan with her because that facilitates the close communication with the high-risk clinic specialists, that is crucial for the management of this situation.

*The patient has presented pregnant and wishes to have a termination. Can that be carried out locally?*

Early first trimester termination usually can be performed with minimal complications but the factors that may make a patient moderate- to high-risk for pregnancy carry the same types of risks for termination. Patients deemed to be low risk can have the procedure locally but it should be performed in a hospital operating room. Moderate- and high-risk patients should obtain a prompt referral to have the procedure at the tertiary center. Certainly any patient who requires termination on medical grounds should be referred urgently to the high-risk center.

*The patient wishes to have a tubal ligation. Can that be carried out locally?*

If the patient has already been seen by the team for a previous assessment and has been considered low risk, it would be appropriate to undertake tubal ligation locally. If there are any doubts, she needs to be referred to the clinic for a risk assessment and plan, in light of the hemodynamic perturbations that may occur during laparoscopy. Similarly, it is important to discuss referral to the clinic for consideration of IUD placement in moderate- and high-risk patients.

*What kind of counseling are these patients getting at the high-risk clinic?*

Depending on their needs, the patients, male and female, are counseled on sexual functioning and contraception. After full assessment, the patients are counseled on their parental and pregnancy risks. This counseling may involve the cardiologist, the obstetrician, the clinical geneticist, the psychologist or psychiatrist, or the advanced practice nurse attached to the clinic. Part of any counseling includes some discussion of patient prognosis. Although there are data for several lesions and clinical situations, new therapies and changing therapies can make the determination of prognosis difficult [5,66]. Any such discussion should be prepared carefully beforehand and presented in a frank but sensitive manner.

*The insurance company refuses to pay for any visits to the high-risk clinic in another city because they claim that the patient can be seen and delivered locally. How can this situation be resolved?*

Some insurance companies or care plans may be reluctant to pay for a referral outside their usual system. Documents such as this one can persuade them that referral of these patients is not just better for the patient and child but crucial for their well being.

## References

[1] Pradat P, Francannet C, Harris JA, et al. The epidemiology of cardiovascular defects, part 1: a study based on data from three large registries of congenital malformations. Pediatr Cardiol 2003;24:195–221.

[2] Gillum RF. Epidemiology of congenital heart disease in the United States. Am Heart J 1994;127: 919–27.

[3] Warnes CA. The adult with congenital heart disease: born to be bad? J Am Coll Cardiol 2005;46:1–8.

[4] Hoyert DL, Mathews TJ, Menacker F, et al. Annual summary of vital statistics: 2004. Pediatrics 2006; 117(1):168–83.

[5] Bhat AH, Sahn DJ. Congenital heart disease never goes away, even when it has been "treated": the adult with congenital heart disease. Curr Opin Pediatr 2004;16:500–7.

[6] Canobbio MM. Health care issues facing adolescents with congenital heart disease. J Pediatr Nurs 2001;16:363–70.

[7] Lane DA, Lip GYH, Millane TA. Congenital heart disease: quality of life in adults with congenital heart disease. Heart 2002;88:71–5.

[8] Kovacs AH, Sears SF, Saidi AS. Biopsychosocial experiences of adults with congenital heart disease: review of the literature. Am Heart J 2005;150: 193–201.

[9] Swan L, Lupton M, Anthony J, et al. Controversies in pregnancy and congenital heart disease. Congenit Heart Dis 2006;1:27–34.

[10] Whittemore R, Hobbins JC, Engle MA. Pregnancy and its outcome in women with and without surgical treatment of congenital heart disease. Am J Cardiol 1982;50:641–51.

[11] Shime J, Mocarski EJM, Hastings D, et al. Congenital heart disease in pregnancy: short- and long-term implications. Am J Obstet Gynecol 1987;156: 313–22.

[12] Abbas AE, Lester SJ, Connolly H. Pregnancy and the cardiovascular system. Int J Cardiol 2005;98: 179–89.

[13] Siu SC, Sermer M, Colman JM, et al. Prospective multicenter study of pregnancy outcomes in women with heart disease. Circulation 2001;104:515–21.

[14] Head CEG, Thorne SA. Congenital heart disease in pregnancy. Postgrad Med J 2005;81:292–8.

[15] Siu SC, Colman JM. Congenital heart disease: heart disease and pregnancy. Heart 2001;85:710–5.

[16] Connolly HM, Warnes CA. Pregnancy and contraception. In: Gatzoulis MA, Webb GD, Daubeney PEF, editors. Diagnosis and management of adult congenital heart disease. London: Churchill Livingstone; 2003.

[17] Hunter S, Robson SC. Adaptation of the maternal heart in pregnancy. Br Heart J 1992;68:540–3.

[18] Varga I, Rigo J, Somos P, et al. Analysis of maternal circulation and renal function in physiologic pregnancies; parallel examinations of the changes in the cardiac output and the glomerular filtration rate. J Maternal-Fetal Med 2000;9: 97–104.

[19] Conrad KP. Mechanisms of renal vasodilation and hyperfiltration during pregnancy. J Soc Gynecol Investig 2004;11:438–48.

[20] Carbillon L, Uzan M, Uzan S. Pregnancy, vascular tone, and maternal hemodynamics: a crucial adaptation. Obstet Gynecol Surv 2000;55:574–81.

[21] Campos O. Doppler echocardiography during pregnancy: physiological and abnormal findings. Echocardiography 1996;13:135–46.

[22] Klein LL, Galan HL. Cardiac disease in pregnancy. Obstet Gynecol Clin N Am 2004;31:429–59.

[23] Duprez D, Kaufman J, Liu Y, et al. Increases in atrial natriuretic peptide after delivery and in the puerperium. Am J Cardiol 1989;64:674–5.

[24] Immer FF, Bansi AG, Immer-Bansi AS, et al. Aortic dissection in pregnancy: analysis of risk factors and outcome. Ann Thorac Surg 2003;76:309–14.

[25] Kelly BA, Bond BC, Poston L. Aortic adaptation to pregnancy: elevated expression of matrix

metalloproteinanes-2 and -3 in rat gestation. Mol Hum Reprod 2004;10:331–7.

[26] Edouard DA, Pannier BM, London GM, et al. Venous and arterial behavior during normal pregnancy. Am J Physiol 1998;274:H1605–12.

[27] Brenner B. Haemostatic changes in pregnancy. Thromb Res 2004;114:409–14.

[28] Uebing A, Steer PJ, Yentis SM, et al. Pregnancy and congenital heart disease. BMJ 2006;332:401–6.

[29] Khairy P, Ouyang DW, Fernandes SM, et al. Pregnancy outcomes in women with congenital heart disease. Circulation 2006;113:517–24.

[30] Niwa K, Siu SC, Webb GD, Gatzoulis MA. Progressive aortic root dilatation in adults after repair of Tetralogy of Fallot. Circulation 2002; 106:1374–8.

[31] Steer PJ. Pregnancy and contraception. In: Gatzoulis M, Swan L, Therrien J, Pantely G, editors. Adult congenital heart disease. Oxford: Blackwell Publishing; 2005. p. 16–35.

[32] Gowda RM, Khan IA, Mehta NJ, et al. Cardiac arrhythmias in pregnancy: clinical and therapeutic considerations. Int J Cardiol 2003;88:129–33.

[33] Shotan A, Ostrzega E, Mehra A, et al. Incidence of arrhythmias in normal pregnancy and relation to palpitations, dizziness, and syncope. Am J Cardiol 1997;79(8):1061–4.

[34] Widerhorn J, Widerhorn ALM, Rahimtoola SH, et al. WPW syndrome during pregnancy: increased incidence of supraventricular arrhythmias. Am Heart J 1992;123:796–8.

[35] Romem A, Romem Y, Katz M, et al. Incidence and characteristics of maternal cardiac arrhythmias during labor. Am J Cardiol 2004;93:931–3.

[36] Campos O, Andrade JL, Bocanegra J, et al. Physiologic multivalvular regurgitation during pregnancy: a longitudinal Doppler echocardiographic study. Int J Cardiol 1993;40:265–72.

[37] Broberg CS, Yentis SM, Steer PJ, et al. Women and congenital heart disease. In: Wenger N, Collins P, editors. Women and heart disease. 2nd edition. New York: Taylor & Francis; 2005. p. 454–71.

[38] De Swiet M, Nelson-Piercy C. Cardiac disease. In: Lewis G, editor. Why mothers die 2000–2002: the sixth report into maternal deaths in the United Kingdom. London: RCOG Press; 2004 Available at:http://www.cemach.org.uk/publications/WMD2000_2002/content.htm. Accessed September 18, 2006.

[39] Siu SC, Colman JM, Sorensen S, et al. Adverse neonatal and cardiac outcomes are more common in pregnant women with cardiac disease. Circulation 2002;105:2179–84.

[40] Avila WA, Rossi EG, Ramires JAF, et al. Pregnancy in patients with heart disease: experience with 1000 cases. Clin Cardiol 2003;26:135–42.

[41] Presbitero P, Somerville J, Stone S, et al. Congenital heart disease: pregnancy in cyanotic congenital heart disease: outcome of mother and fetus. Circulation 1994;89:2673–6.

[42] Georgieff MK. Intrauterine growth retardation and subsequent somatic growth and neurodevelopment. J Pediatr 1998;133:3–5.

[43] Brodszki J, Lanne T, Marsal K, et al. Pediatric cardiology: impaired vascular growth in late adolescence after intrauterine growth restriction. Circulation 2005;111:2623–8.

[44] Barker DJ. Early growth and cardiovascular disease. Arch Dis Child 1999;80:305–10.

[45] Romano-Zelekha O, Hirsh R, Blieden L, et al. The risk for congenital heart defects in offspring of individuals with congenital heart defects. Clin Genet 2001;59:325–9.

[46] Burn J, Brennan P, Little J, et al. Recurrence risks in offspring of adults with major heart defects: results from first cohort of British collaborative study. Lancet 1998;351:311–6.

[47] Lupton M, Oteng-Ntim E, Ayida G, et al. Cardiac disease in pregnancy. Curr Opin Obstet Gynecol 2002;14:137–43.

[48] Renforth GL, Wilson DI. Adults with congenital heart disease: a genetic perspective. In: Gatzoulis MA, Webb GD, Daubeney PEF, editors. Diagnosis and management of adult congenital heart disease. London: Churchill Livingstone; 2003. p. 19–24.

[49] Nora JJ. From generational studies to a multilevel genetic-environmental interaction. J Am Coll Cardiol 1994;23:1468–71.

[50] Bassett AS, Chow EWC, Husted J, et al. Clinical features of 78 adults with 22q11 deletion syndrome. Am J Med Genet 2005;138A:307–13.

[51] Carvalho JS. Early prenatal diagnosis of major congenital heart defects. Curr Opin Obstet Gynecol 2001;13:155–9.

[52] Canobbio MM, Perloff JK, Rapkin AJ. Gynecological health of females with congenital heart disease. Int J Cardiol 2005;98:379–87.

[53] Reid GJ, Irvine MJ, McCrindle BW, et al. Prevalence and correlates of successful transfer from pediatric to adult health care among a cohort of young adults with complex congenital heart defects. Pediatrics 2004;113:197–205.

[54] Kafka H, Uemura H, Gatzoulis MA. Surgical and catheter intervention during pregnancy in patients with heart disease. In: Steer P, Gatzoulis MA, Baker P, editors. Cardiac disease and pregnancy. London: RCOG Press; 2006. p. 95–128.

[55] Leonard H, O'Sullivan J, Hunter S. Family planning requirements in the adult congenital heart disease clinic. Heart 1996;76:60–2.

[56] ACOG Committee Opinion No. 299. Guidelines for diagnostic imaging during pregnancy. Obstet Gynecol 2004;104:647–51.

[57] Leyendecker JR, Gorengaut V, Brown JJ. MR imaging of maternal diseases of the abdomen and pelvis during pregnancy and the immediate postpartum period. Radiographics 2004;24:1301–16.

[58] James PR. Cardiovascular disease. Best Pract Res Clin Obstet Gynaecol 2001;15:903–11.

[59] Elkayam U. Pregnancy through a prosthetic heart valve. J Am Coll Cardiol 1999;33:1642–5.

[60] Bates SM, Greer IA, Hirsh J, et al. Use of antithrombotic agents during pregnancy. Chest 2004;126: 627S–44S.

[61] Qasqas SA, McPherson C, Frishman WH, et al. Cardiovascular pharmacotherapeutic considerations during pregnancy and lactation. Cardiol Rev 2004; 12:201–21.

[62] Thorne SA. Pregnancy in heart disease. Heart 2004; 90:450–6.

[63] Magee LA. Antihypertensives. Best Pract Res Clin Obstet Gynaecol 2001;15:827–45.

[64] Ro A, Frishman WH. Peripartum cardiomyopathy. Cardiol Rev 2006;14:35–42.

[65] Greenberg SS, Lancaster JR, Xie J, et al. Effects of NO synthase inhibitors, arginine-deficient diet, and amiloride in pregnant rats. Am J Physiol 1997;273: R1031–45.

[66] Vonder Muhl I, Cumming G, Gatzoulis MA. Risky business: insuring adults with congenital heart disease. Eur Heart J 2003;24:1595–600.

ELSEVIER
SAUNDERS

Cardiol Clin 24 (2006) 607–618

CARDIOLOGY
CLINICS

# The Role of the Psychologist in Adult Congenital Heart Disease

Adrienne H. Kovacs, PhD[a],*, Candice Silversides, MD[b],
Arwa Saidi, MB, BCh[c], Samuel F. Sears, PhD[d]

[a]Cardiac Psychology, Division of Cardiology, University Health Network, 399 Bathurst Street,
1-West-414, Toronto, ON M5T 2N2, Canada
[b]Division of Cardiology, University Health Network, University of Toronto,
Toronto General Hospital, 585 University Avenue, 5N-521, Toronto, ON M5G 2N2, Canada
[c]Departments of Pediatrics and Internal Medicine, University of Florida, PO Box 100296,
1600 SW Archer Road, Gainesville, FL 32610, USA
[d]Department of Clinical and Health Psychology, College of Public Health and Health Professions,
University of Florida, Box 100165 UFHSC, 1600 SW Archer Road, Gainesville, FL 32610, USA

Due to diagnostic, surgical, interventional, and pharmacologic advances, it is estimated that up to 95% of infants born with congenital heart defects will reach adulthood [1]. There are now more adults than children living with congenital heart disease [2], but there exists a less than ideal capacity to manage adults in pediatric or adult cardiology clinics. Adult congenital heart disease (ACHD) patients are at an increased risk of late cardiac complications including arrhythmias, endocarditis, congestive heart failure, and pulmonary vascular disease. The effects of chronic illness, multiple surgical admissions, and hospitalization in childhood, adolescence, and adulthood can have a significant impact on the psychological well-being of these patients. The evidence for psychological distress in impacting health outcomes and quality of life (QOL) across cardiac patient populations is now considered by some as "clear and convincing" [3]. Psychological distress is common following cardiac diagnosis, with approximately 20% to 50% of patients reporting adjustment difficulties [4]. Therefore, in addition to monitoring and treating the medical sequelae, it is important to recognize and manage the potential psychosocial consequences of growing up with congenital heart disease [5,6]. International working groups have emphasized the inclusion of specialized mental health care for ACHD [7–9]. The summary document of the 32nd Bethesda Conference ("Care of the Adult with Congenital Heart Disease") included the following statement: "The emotional health of adults with [congenital heart disease] should be a priority in the overall care of this patient population" [7]. Similarly, the Task Force on the Management of Grown Up Congenital Heart Disease of the European Society of Cardiology stated, "The specialist service for grown-ups with congenital heart disease must provide support for the many psychosocial problems in this population" [9].

In this article, the authors review the evidence that patients who have ACHD have special and unique psychosocial needs and discuss ways in which psychologists can be integrated into multidisciplinary ACHD care teams. The psychosocial adjustment and QOL issues observed in adults who have grown up with congenital heart defects are reviewed. Three professional domains in which clinical health psychologists can contribute to an ACHD team—provision of clinical services, multidisciplinary research, and professional education—are discussed in detail. Finally, considerations for introducing or increasing the presence of psychology in ACHD teams are presented.

* Corresponding author.
*E-mail address:* adrienne.kovacs@uhn.on.ca
(A.H. Kovacs).

## Psychosocial adjustment in adult congenital heart disease

### Psychological functioning

The increasing number of published studies evaluating the psychological aspects of ACHD reflects the growing recognition of the potential emotional and behavioral implications of growing up with a serious medical condition. In general, ACHD patients are at greater risk of psychological difficulties than adults who have not lived with chronic medical conditions [10–13]. Based on studies that employed clinical interview methodologies, it is estimated that 35% to 79% of ACHD patients meet diagnostic criteria for a psychiatric diagnosis [11,13]. Of note, this figure of 35% was observed in a sample of ACHD patients deemed "well adjusted" by their medical teams. There are, however, European data suggestive of favorable psychological adjustment among ACHD patients compared with healthy peers [14–17].

Conflicting results might reflect variation in measurement tools, study populations, and methodologic approaches associated with self-report versus interview assessments. ACHD patients might under-report psychological symptoms on self-report measures as a reflection of denial and high achievement motivation [14,16]. Clinical interviews likely offer the most accurate picture of psychological adjustment. Reported differences in psychological adjustment might also reflect sociocultural differences in the long-term care of individuals who have chronic medical conditions [5]. Individuals from countries with universal access and stronger mental health care systems might report more positive health expectations or experiences.

Compared with the general population, it appears that the proportion of ACHD patients experiencing psychological distress is elevated. Risk factors related to psychological difficulties in this population have been studied, and it has been demonstrated that younger patients tend to have more psychological problems than older patients and women appear to have more psychological difficulties than men [18,19]. Results investigating the impact of medical variables are inconsistent. Studies by Brandhagen and colleagues [10] and Utens and colleagues [14,15] found that disease variables were unrelated to psychological symptoms, whereas other studies found that disease severity was related to psychological symptoms [13,18]. Van Rijen and coworkers [18]

found that significant medical predictors of patient-reported behavioral and emotional problems included low maximal exercise capacity, physician-imposed restrictions, and negative personal experiences with scarring. Popelova and colleagues [12] found that depressive symptoms were associated with poorer functional state. Collectively, these studies suggest that functional status might be a stronger predictor of psychological health than disease severity. Although psychologists obviously cannot impact the sex or age of a patient, other factors including depressive symptoms, perception of scarring, and even functional status (eg, reflecting improved exercise capacity) are often amenable to change.

### Quality of life

A complete understanding of the experience of growing up with a congenital heart defect includes not only traditional markers of psychological maladjustment (ie, anxiety and depression) but also health-related QOL. QOL has emerged as an end point of interest because it reflects a patient's life satisfaction and ability to function in a variety of life domains including physical, social, emotional, and work-related. Some researchers believe it is embodied in the approach of the biopsychosocial model of health in which biologic, psychological, and social functioning are interdependent [20]. QOL, however, should not be equated with health status. Moons and colleagues [21] defined QOL as "the degree of overall life satisfaction that is positively or negatively influenced by individuals' perception of certain aspects of life important to them, including matters both related and unrelated to health." Moons and coworkers [22] described a "paradigm shift" in the conceptualization of the QOL of ACHD patients, such that QOL is most accurately understood through examination of domains deemed important to an individual patient, rather than through the administration of standardized questionnaires. Among ACHD patients, the most important determinants of an individual's QOL are family, job/education, friends, health, and leisure time [22].

Although some researchers have concluded that QOL in patients who have congenital heart disease is poorer compared with healthy peers [23–26], others have not [27–29]. Poor QOL in the ACHD population has been linked with (1) clinical variables (cyanosis, orthopedic problems); (2) social variables (lower level of educational attainment, age, social impediments); and (3) psychological variables (negative thoughts) [28,30,31]. Saliba and colleagues [28] detected poorer QOL in cyanotic patients compared with their noncyanotic peers. Simko and McGinnis [32] found that individuals who had acyanotic defects had better QOL than those who had single-ventricle physiology. Ternestedt and coworkers [33] noted that individuals who had tetralogy of Fallot reported better QOL than individuals who had atrial septal defects, an unexpected finding given that atrial septal defects are generally considered a more benign cardiac lesion. There are data, however, that suggest that indices of functional status might be stronger predictors of QOL than the severity of the initial cardiac diagnoses [34]. For example, Rose and colleagues [26] observed that objective cardiopulmonary functioning strongly impacted cardiac complaints and the physical component of health-related QOL. Psychological intervention can target functional status through the promotion of healthy lifestyle behaviors including exercise, diet, and adherence to medical regimens.

*Social adjustment*

Some individuals experience difficult familial and peer interactions as a result of growing up with congenital heart defects. Approximately one fourth of ACHD patients describe parental overprotection in childhood and adolescence [10,35]. ACHD patients are more likely to live with their parents than their healthy peers [36]. "Feeling different" and body image concerns are common to many adolescents and young adults living with congenital heart disease [11,37,38]. Horner and colleagues [11] observed a pattern of pervasive denial during their interviews with 29 ACHD patients. It was common for their ACHD interviewees to reveal difficulties with childhood and adolescent social interactions only after extensive questioning. Many of these interviewees also recalled coping with negative childhood interactions by wearing "a happy face" and behaving as though "everything was fine." As adolescents who have congenital heart disease progress into adulthood, they are presented with a new set of challenges. Difficulties obtaining employment and health insurance can be particularly frustrating [12,30,39]. In addition, issues surrounding contraception, pregnancy, and parenthood require extra consideration for many ACHD patients [40]. Psychologists can provide supportive and cognitive-behavioral therapy for these difficult issues (eg, managing social anxiety, managing stress, strategies for discussing sensitive issues with one's medical team).

*Limitations of current research*

There is a sample bias when studying a restricted group of individuals. ACHD patients in these studies are typically those who (1) receive follow-up care for a congenital heart defect, (2) receive their care at a facility with a program of research, (3) are not excluded based on cognitive functioning, and (4) consent to participate in research studies. It is unfortunate that most individuals born with heart defects do not receive specialized ACHD care [41]; therefore, study results cannot necessarily be generalized to the entire population of ACHD patients. We have no way of knowing whether the psychosocial health of ACHD patients who are lost to cardiology follow-up (or who present to smaller cardiology clinics at which research is not conducted) is better or worse than that of study participants; however, the authors believe that the conclusions can be generalized to patients who present at ACHD specialty centers.

*Need for specialized care*

There is a growing recognition of the biopsychosocial implications of growing up with congenital heart disease. In addition to specialized assessment and treatment of the biomedical sequelae of cardiac defects, the psychosocial well-being of this population deserves specialized mental health care. With assessment and psychotherapeutic techniques, psychologists are able to provide emotional support and specific strategies to maximize psychological well-being.

Psychologists typically have doctorates in philosophy (PhD), education (EdD), or psychology (PsyD). Psychologists receive specialized training in assessment; case conceptualization; individual, family, or group psychotherapy; professional ethics; research design; and statistical analysis. Strategies of a cognitive-behavioral psychologist include worry management, thought restructuring, relaxation training, behavioral activation, and communication skills training. Psychologists who have health psychology experience are aware of the relationship between physical health and psychological health and are able to tailor the aforementioned strategies to assist individuals in managing their illness experience. They are also able to "normalize" patient experiences (versus adopting a pathologic conceptualization of emotional responses to illness). Psychiatrists, by comparison, are medical doctors and are more strongly associated with a biologic approach to mental health. Psychotropic medication can be an important component of treatment for many

ACHD patients; however, it is not a replacement for psychotherapy ("talk therapy"), and some ACHD patients are reluctant to add to a complex medication regimen. Collectively, psychology and psychiatry can collaborate to provide optimal mental health treatment for ACHD patients.

### Roles of psychologists in adult congenital heart disease

*Provision of clinical services*

The 32nd Bethesda Conference stated, "Appropriate screening and referral sources for [mental health] treatment should be available at all regional ACHD centers" [7]. Similarly, the Canadian Consensus document stated that consultation with psychology/psychiatry is indicated to "facilitate optimal functioning," to address clinical and subclinical depression and anxiety, and to enhance adjustment to illness exacerbations and hospitalizations [8]. The European Task Force also emphasized the importance of support for the psychological difficulties of ACHD patients [9]. Despite these recommendations, there is underdiagnosis and undertreatment of psychosocial concerns in ACHD patients [13]; therefore, clinical health psychologists have clear potential to be important members of ACHD teams. Psychologists are able to diagnose psychiatric disorders and provide treatment or to assist with referrals to other mental health professionals when appropriate.

Symptoms of mood and anxiety disorders are two of the more obvious indications for referral to a psychologist. In a cardiology setting, such referrals are particularly warranted because psychosocial factors are associated with the onset of coronary artery disease and increased cardiac mortality [42–44]. For example, depression following myocardial infarction has been linked with a 2- to 2.5-fold increase in cardiovascular events or mortality [45]. Additional specific indications for referral to a psychologist working with an ACHD team are provided in Box 1 and then discussed in detail.

*Psychological distress*
*Difficulties coping with medical condition.* Although there is a tendency for some patients to consider themselves "cured," the reality is that many require lifelong medical follow-up [1]. Research suggests that functional status is more strongly related to QOL than cardiac defect severity [34]. It can be a significant psychological setback when patients unexpectedly experience decrements

---

**Box 1. Common indications for referral to psychology**

Psychological distress
    Difficulties coping with medical
        condition
    Cardiac anxiety
    Patient mortality concerns

Medical treatment–related issues
    Treatment decision making
    Surgical preparation
    Adjustment to cardiac devices

Psychosocial difficulties
    Family and peer concerns
    Difficult pediatric–adult transitions

Healthy lifestyle concerns
    Behavioral modification
    Maximizing adherence

Developmental/neurocognitive issues

---

in their functional status or learn that further medical or surgical intervention is advised. Horner and colleagues [11] reported that many of their interviewees were angry when cardiac complications developed in adulthood after years of relative stability. Although this article focuses on the experiences of adults who have grown up with congenital heart disease, some ACHD patients do not learn of their cardiac defect until adulthood. These individuals may be ill prepared to cope with the impact of this new diagnosis and its implications. Psychologists can provide emotional support and cognitive-behavioral strategies to manage anger and health-related stressors.

*Cardiac anxiety.* Heart-focused anxiety refers to the fear of cardiac sensations and events (eg, increased heart rate) because of presumed negative consequences [46]. Clinical experience suggests that this is more common after individuals are informed that their cardiac condition has worsened or that they require follow-up procedures or closer cardiac monitoring. Patients who have higher cardiac anxiety tend to pay greater attention to cardiac sensations and avoid certain activities they fear will trigger cardiac symptoms [46]. For example, among a sample of patients who had implantable cardioverter defibrillators (ICDs), patients who had panic disorder were more likely to report attempts to pay attention to bodily changes to avoid being surprised by their next shocks and the belief that they could perceive heartbeat irregularities [47]. Utens and colleagues [15] hypothesized that increased somatic complaints among ACHD patients might reflect their heightened alertness to bodily symptoms. This increased somatic hypersensitivity might correspond to an increased risk of psychological stress, particularly anxiety. Rietveld and coworkers [48] found that compared with healthy comparison peers, ACHD patients were more likely to be distracted by their heart beats during a concentration task and were less accurate at estimating their heart rate during another task. Unexpectedly, in this sample, ACHD patients did not report more anxiety associated with audible heartbeats than healthy comparison peers. Psychologists can assist individuals who have cardiac anxiety by way of psychoeducation and the provision of strategies selected to reduce excessive self-monitoring of cardiac symptoms and to promote engagement in avoided activities.

*Patient mortality concerns.* The psychosocial concerns of ACHD patients do not remain static throughout their lifetimes. Individuals who have chronic medical conditions develop an "illness career" that varies in response to several factors including changes in health and interactions with health care professionals [49]. Certain situations result in increased patient awareness of mortality (ie, changes in cardiac status, including but not limited to being informed of terminal status). In this difficult stage of life, it is important that patients, if they choose, are able to clearly discuss their concerns and fears with supportive individuals. Patients may be reluctant to disclose their concerns to physicians for a variety of reasons, including not wanting to "burden" their physicians with nonmedical concerns. Patients might also be cautious to reveal their fears and concerns to family members who are already distressed by the situation. Psychologists can assist these individuals during this difficult time by providing emotional support, discussing anticipatory grief, and sharing strategies to communicate most effectively with medical teams and loved ones.

### Medical treatment–related issues
*Treatment decision making.* Cardiac patients are often asked to make difficult medical decisions. For example, they might be recommended to undergo invasive cardiac procedures, many of which have relatively high risks of complications.

They may have difficulties understanding medical recommendations and respond with exaggerated fears. Patients may benefit from additional support or counseling to be able to commit to these complex care decisions. For any difficult decision, it is important that depression or anxiety does not distort patient judgment [50,51]. Psychologists can evaluate the psychological functioning of individuals who are making difficult decisions. They can also assist patients in the decision-making process (eg, with a decisional balance exercise in which the pros and cons of options are thoroughly reviewed).

*Surgical preparation.* Greater presurgical anxiety is associated with more complicated and slower surgical recovery [52]. Psychological factors can influence surgical recovery through endocrine and immune functioning and behavioral mechanisms (including smoking and poor diet) [52]. Meta-analytic studies indicate that psychological preparation for surgery and psychoeducational interventions can positively impact outcomes including psychological distress, pain, and surgical recovery [53,54]. Psychologists can offer surgical preparation techniques (including stress management and imagery) that have proved effective in the reduction of anxiety for cardiac patients undergoing surgical procedures [55].

*Adjustment to cardiac devices.* The use of ICDs is an increasing treatment for ACHD patients at risk for sudden cardiac death [56]; however, this life-saving technology is not without psychosocial impact. Although in general, ICDs appear equal or better than antiarrhythmic medications in terms of their impact on patient QOL [57–60], they lead to significant psychological distress for many device recipients. Approximately 13% to 38% of recipients experience diagnosable levels of anxiety, and significant depression is observed in 24% to 33% of recipients [61]. Younger age and greater frequency of ICD firings appear to be the strongest risk factors for psychological distress [61]. The provision of ICD-specific education and cognitive-behavioral strategies by psychologists can enhance the confidence and QOL of ICD recipients [62].

### Psychosocial difficulties
*Family and peer concerns.* As outlined earlier, parental overprotection and difficult peer interactions are common among ACHD patients. Furthermore, childhood and adolescent experiences with peers and family are not always easily

forgotten in adulthood. Some ACHD patients benefit from social skills training. Others benefit from learning communication strategies to exert increased independence with family members or to be more involved in their health care. These are two specific examples in which psychologists can provide interventions to enhance social well-being.

*Difficult pediatric–adult transitions.* The transition from pediatric to adult health care can be tumultuous for many ACHD patients (see the article by Webb and Reiss found elsewhere in this issue). Many adolescents who have congenital heart disease do not successfully transition to adult care [63]. Although successful transition begins in the pediatric setting, psychologists working in ACHD can provide individual consultation to patients experiencing a difficult transition (eg, offering strategies to empower patients to assume increased control over their cardiac management). In addition, psychologists can contribute to a formalized transition program. For example, the Toronto Congenital Cardiac Centre for Adults currently offers transition nights for 17- and 18-year-old pediatric patients before their first visit to the center. A psychologist attends these meetings to proactively discuss transition issues with patients and families.

### Healthy lifestyle concerns
*Behavioral modification.* A healthy lifestyle including a well-balanced diet and an individually appropriate level of physical activity is important for all individuals but even more so for those who have cardiac conditions. Dusseldorp and colleagues [64] conducted a meta-analysis of psychoeducation programs for individuals who had coronary artery disease and concluded that such interventions had a positive impact on healthy lifestyle behaviors (eg, body weight, diet, exercise habits) and resulted in reduced cardiac mortality and recurrence of myocardial infarction. Although there are no studies examining the impact of psychoeducation targeting heart-healthy behaviors for ACHD patients, it is assumed that such education is beneficial. It is unfortunate that ACHD patients are usually less likely to engage in physical activity [65]. Psychologists can provide behavioral strategies for the adoption and maintenance of a physician-approved physical activity regimen that empowers patients to exercise control over their condition.

*Maximizing adherence.* Kulkarni and colleagues [66] noted that CAD patients often stop medications within 1 year of their prescription. They also found that poorer adherence to a cardiovascular medication regimen was linked to a number of factors including lower educational attainment, older age, greater number of medications prescribed, and poorer mental health [66]. Depression is strongly linked to nonadherence to medical treatments [67] and has been associated with nonadherence to the prescribed behavioral and lifestyle modifications in postmyocardial infarction patients [68]. In a sample of heart failure patients, depression has also been associated with patient-reported difficulty taking medications as directed by physicians [69]. Psychologists can provide strategies that target depressive symptoms and nonadherence concerns concurrently.

### Developmental/neurocognitive issues
Neuropsychologic assessment in individuals who have congenital heart disease can help to detect cerebral dysfunction in the absence of anatomic alterations in the brain and to evaluate the cognitive impact of disease [70]. Neurocognitive deficits are associated with certain genetic disorders (eg, Down syndrome) and sequelae from ischemia/hypoxia and pediatric cardiopulmonary bypass. A review of the impact of chronic or intermittent hypoxia on cognition in childhood indicated adverse impacts on cognitive, behavioral, and academic outcomes [71]. The impact of cardiac defects on cognitive and academic performance may persist even after cardiac surgery [72]. In a study of individuals who were operated on during childhood for tetralogy of Fallot, the most common cognitive deficits were exhibited in tasks that demanded executive functioning, problem solving, and planning (rather than memory, learning, or attention); many of these patients also reported a lower than normal level of academic achievement [73]. In another study, approximately one fourth of ACHD patients had participated in special education [16]. A thorough review of the neurocognitive deficits associated with specific congenital heart defects is beyond the scope of this article, but excellent summaries are available [70,74]. Neuropsychologists can prove to be especially valuable in the assessment of neurocognitive functioning of children, adolescents, and adults who have congenital heart defects.

### Multidisciplinary research

As stated earlier, psychologists receive extensive training in research design and statistical analysis during their graduate training and are therefore able to contribute to the overall research agenda of an ACHD team. Box 2 indicates potential areas of collaborative research. In all areas of ACHD patient research (biomedical or psychosocial), multicenter studies are recommended. To truly increase our understanding of ACHD patient experiences, collaboration between health care teams at different centers is crucial.

*Development of adult congenital heart disease–specific measures*

Within the cardiac psychology and nursing literature, there are specific measures targeting different subgroups of patients, including those who have angina, heart failure, ICDs, and so forth. Therefore, it is generally accepted that the patient experience can differ across cardiac conditions. American and European guidelines call for the creation of psychosocial measures specifically developed for the ACHD patient population [7,9]. Kamphuis and colleagues [75] developed and validated a specific assessment tool for ACHD patients that has three subscales pertaining to problems associated with physical symptoms, cardiac monitoring and treatment (eg, echocardiography, taking blood, hospital admission), and worries. Additional ACHD-specific measures should be developed that address the unique concerns of this patient population. For example, just as the left ventricular ejection fraction is generally less meaningful for ACHD patients, psychosocial measures designed for adults who have acquired cardiac disease do not capture the full ACHD patient experience (eg, transition from pediatric to adult cardiology care, chronic cyanosis, and so forth). Health professionals (including psychologists) who have knowledge of the unique ACHD patient experiences are best able to create and evaluate such measures.

*Longitudinal psychosocial assessment*

There are few prospective studies examining the psychosocial adjustment of ACHD patients;

**Box 2. Areas of research**

Development of ACHD-specific measures
Longitudinal psychosocial assessment
Evaluation of psychological interventions
Evaluation of medical interventions
Relationship between mental and physical health

most research has used a cross-sectional design. Longitudinal studies, by definition, would allow us to monitor the psychosocial functioning of ACHD over time to better understand the impact of the transition from pediatric to adult care, changing cardiac status, and general aging experiences of ACHD patients.

*Evaluation of psychological interventions*

Despite an increasing awareness of the psychosocial concerns of the ACHD patient population, there are no published trials of psychological interventions for ACHD patients [76]. One practical consideration is the fact that many individuals attending ACHD outpatient clinics travel quite a distance to attend clinics. For this reason, "creative solutions for counseling patients in groups or those who live a far distance away should be developed" [7]. Interventions provided by telephone or over the Internet might be most realistic for many ACHD patients.

*Evaluation of medical interventions*

The impact of surgical and interventional procedures is not limited to cardiac anatomy. Successful outcomes include improvements in functional status and health-related QOL. Biomedical and psychosocial outcomes should be investigated to demonstrate the effectiveness of medical treatment. The summary document of the 32nd Bethesda Conference recommended investigating the physical and psychosocial impact of regular follow-up [7], which illustrates the importance of multidisciplinary research such that physician, nursing, and psychology staff collaborate to best understand the biopsychosocial experience of medical treatment.

*Relationship between mental and physical health*

In the previous paragraph, research examining the impact of medical intervention on psychosocial functioning was recommended. It is equally important to examine the influence of psychological factors on physical functioning. Coronary artery disease literature suggests that the relationship between psychosocial status and cardiac outcome might be mediated by physiologic mechanisms including alteration of catecholamine activity, inflammatory responses, and impaired cardiovascular reactivity. Behavioral pathways linking psychosocial health and cardiac outcome include adherence to prescribed treatments and the adoption of healthy lifestyle behaviors. It is now time to investigate ways in which psychosocial factors might influence medical outcomes of

ACHD patients (eg, surgical recovery, heart functioning, disease progression, and so forth). Again, this line of research demands multidisciplinary collaboration between medicine, nursing, and psychology.

### Professional education

The third area in which psychologists can contribute to ACHD care teams involves the education of medical trainees (including nursing trainees) and student psychologists. As defined by current guidelines, competency as a level 2 or level 3 ACHD specialist includes knowledge of psychosocial aspects of adolescence, the transition to adulthood, experience with lifestyle counseling, and advocacy [7,9]. These training guidelines suggest that exposure to other professionals including psychologists is important during training. Education for cardiology residents and fellows, staff cardiologists, and nurses can occur formally (eg, presentation at professional meetings, rounds, case conferences) and informally (eg, casual questions/interactions). Box 3 presents the more formal teaching topics for medical trainees and psychologists.

### Increased psychosocial awareness

Kovacs and colleagues [5] provided a list of six clinical strategies to maximize psychosocial care of ACHD patients. This list included the increased psychosocial awareness of cardiologists working within ACHD. Psychologists are the most qualified individuals to educate physicians and nursing staff regarding the psychosocial experiences of ACHD due to their knowledge of relevant research and clinical experiences; case studies can often be more poignant and memorable than data summaries. Psychologists emphasize the diversity of the patient experience. Not all ACHD patients experience significant psychological distress, and triggers of distress vary greatly between individuals.

---

**Box 3. Formal teaching topics**

Increased psychosocial awareness
Indications for referral to a mental health
  practitioner
Physician–patient communication skills
  training
Training psychologists to work in ACHD

---

### Indications for referral to a mental health practitioner

Psychology referrals might be patient initiated or physician initiated. ACHD patients occasionally inquire directly about mental health treatment; at other times, physicians broach this topic with their patients. In such situations, it is imperative that referral to psychology (or psychiatry) be made with the patient's knowledge. Referrals should not be automatic when a patient bursts into tears during a clinic appointment; it is important for the physician or nurse to inquire whether this reflects ongoing psychological distress or is a transient reaction to a stressful medical situation. It is also important to clarify appropriate referral indications with the particular psychologist or psychologists working with an ACHD team. These referral indications might include those presented earlier in this article; however, there might be situations in which it is more appropriate to refer to other mental health professionals including neuropsychologists, psychiatrists, and mental health professionals who have experience in eating disorders, family therapy, and specific psychiatric disorders. For example, individuals who have 22q11 deletion syndrome have significantly higher rates of psychotic disorders and should be evaluated by a psychiatrist [77]. Substance abuse is another example of a problem that is best treated by individuals who specialize in this area. Among ACHD patients, substance abuse is of particular concern because it has been linked to unsuccessful transitions from pediatric to adult health care [63].

### Physician–patient communication skills training

Patients consistently report that they want to be heard by their medical team. Therefore, improving physician–patient communication skills can be very beneficial. A number of situations exist in which such communication can be especially tricky, including delivering "bad news" and proactive discussions of challenging issues such as pregnancy and medical prognosis. Patient participation in medical consultations can be enhanced through physician behaviors [78]. For interested readers, Street and colleagues [78] provided a sample of physician statements intended to build partnerships with patients and increase patient participation. Psychologists can educate physician and nursing staff with regard to the importance of effective communication and patient participation in their medical care. They can also present strategies for improving physician–patient communication.

*Training psychologists to work in ACHD*

It is important that psychologists working in ACHD strive to educate interested student psychologists at various stages in their training (including graduate school practica, predoctoral internships, and postdoctoral fellowships). The 32nd Bethesda Conference emphasized the importance of developing training programs for nonphysician staff including psychologists [7]. Similarly, the 1996 Canadian Consensus Conference on Adult Congenital Heart Disease suggested that an ideal supraregional ACHD referral center would establish and evaluate ongoing training criteria for cardiologists, surgeons, and associated staff including psychologists [8]. Psychologists working with ACHD patients should strive to educate student psychologists, with the ultimate goal of increasing the number of psychologists who have ACHD-specific training.

**Considerations for integrating psychology**

A number of factors impact the level of involvement of a psychologist in an ACHD team:

*The overall commitment of an adult congenital heart disease team to the psychosocial concerns of their patients*

It is difficult to ignore the research findings that suggest that ACHD patients are at increased risk of psychosocial difficulties compared with individuals who did not grow up with lifelong medical conditions. Recognition of psychosocial concerns, however, does not imply a commitment to address these concerns. It can require significant effort and financial support to introduce a psychologist into the ACHD care team.

*The size of the adult congenital heart disease program*

A larger ACHD program with a number of physicians and nurses may be better able to support a more involved psychologist. Such a program might support a "clinic within a clinic" model in which psychologists see patients during the outpatient cardiology clinics and are available for "on-the-spot consultation" [5]. For a smaller program, however, it may be more reasonable to identify psychologists in the medical facility or community for clinical referrals or research collaboration. Regardless of the level of involvement, it is important to establish a plan for integration of the psychologist into the care team (eg,

education seminars for trainees and staff, attendance at clinical rounds).

*The availability of psychologists who have specialized cardiac experience*

Ideally, it is desirable to work with a psychologist who has specialized ACHD experience; however, few psychologists currently have this experience. It is more realistic to seek connections with psychologists who have experience in health psychology and, preferably, specialized training in a cardiac setting.

*Reimbursement for psychology*

In the United States, many ACHD patients do not have health insurance that covers psychological services. In the Canadian province of Ontario, outpatient psychology is not covered in the provincial health plan. Thus, in North America, it is very unlikely that psychologists working with ACHD patients will be adequately reimbursed under a fee-for-service system. Similarly, the Psychosocial Working Group of the Association for European Pediatric Cardiology has acknowledged difficulties with reimbursement for mental health professionals and reported that psychosocial professionals are typically funded through mixed resources [79]. It is therefore likely that the inclusion of a psychologist into an ACHD team would require a strong financial commitment from the ACHD center.

**Summary**

The recognition and management of psychosocial difficulties among ACHD patients deserves increased attention. Working groups from Europe and North America have emphasized the inclusion of specialized mental health care for ACHD patients. There are a number of ways in which psychologists can be integrated into multidisciplinary ACHD care teams. These include the provision of clinical services, collaboration in a multidisciplinary research ream, and the provision of professional education to trainees in cardiology, nursing, and psychology. Barriers exist to the integration of psychologists, including the availability of individuals who have specialized cardiac psychology experience and concerns relating to financial reimbursement. Integration of psychologists requires a strong commitment from an ACHD center but would positively impact the lives of ACHD patients.

# References

[1] Warnes CA. The adult with congenital heart disease: born to be bad? J Am Coll Cardiol 2005;46(1): 1–8.

[2] Webb G. Improving the care of Canadian adults with congenital heart disease. Can J Cardiol 2005; 21(10):833–8.

[3] Rozanski A, Blumenthal JA, Kaplan J. Impact of psychological factors on the pathogenesis of cardiovascular disease and implications for therapy. Circulation 1999;99(16):2192–217.

[4] Carney RM, Freedland KE, Sheline YI, et al. Depression and coronary heart disease: a review for cardiologists. Clin Cardiol 1997;20(3):196–200.

[5] Kovacs AH, Sears SF, Saidi A. Biopsychosocial experiences of adults with congenital heart disease: review of the literature. Am Heart J 2005;150(2): 193–201.

[6] Moons P, De Geest S, Budts W. Comprehensive care for adults with congenital heart disease: expanding roles for nurses. Eur J Cardiovasc Nurs 2002;1(1): 23–8.

[7] Care of the Adult with Congenital Heart Disease. Presented at the 32nd Bethesda Conference. Bethesda, Maryland, October 2–3, 2000. J Am Coll Cardiol 2001;37:1161–98.

[8] Connelly MS, Webb GD, Somerville J, et al. Canadian Consensus Conference on Adult Congenital Heart Disease 1996. Can J Cardiol 1998;14(3): 395–452.

[9] The Task Force on the Management of Grown Up Congenital Heart Disease, European Society of Cardiology, ESC Committee for Practice Guidelines. Management of grown up congenital heart disease. Eur Heart J 2003;24(11):1035–84.

[10] Brandhagen DJ, Feldt RH, Williams DE. Long-term psychological implications of congenital heart disease: a 25-year follow-up. Mayo Clin Proc 1991; 66(5):474–9.

[11] Horner T, Liberthson R, Jellinek MS. Psychosocial profile of adults with complex congenital heart disease. Mayo Clin Proc 2000;75(1):31–6.

[12] Popelova J, Slavik Z, Skovranek J. Are cyanosed adults with congenital cardiac malformations depressed? Cardiol Young 2001;11(4):379–84.

[13] Bromberg JI, Beasley PJ, D'Angelo EJ, et al. Depression and anxiety in adults with congenital heart disease: a pilot study. Heart Lung 2003;32(2): 105–10.

[14] Utens EM, Verhulst FC, Erdman RA, et al. Psychosocial functioning of young adults after surgical correction for congenital heart disease in childhood: a follow up study. J Psychosom Res 1994;38(7): 745–58.

[15] Utens EM, Bieman HJ, Verhulst FC, et al. Psychopathology in young adults with congenital heart disease: follow up results. Eur Heart J 1998;19(4): 647–51.

[16] Van Rijen EH, Utens EM, Roos-Hesselink JW, et al. Psychosocial functioning of the adult with congenital heart disease: a 20–33 years follow up. Eur Heart J 2003;24(7):673–83.

[17] Cox D, Lewis G, Stuart G, et al. A cross-sectional study of the prevalence of psychopathology in adults with congenital heart disease. J Psychosom Res 2002;52(2):65–8.

[18] van Rijen EH, Utens EM, Roos-Hesselink JW, et al. Medical predictors for psychopathology in adults with operated congenital heart disease. Eur Heart J 2004;25(18):1605–13.

[19] van Rijen EH, Utens EM, Roos-Hesselink JW, et al. Longitudinal development of psychopathology in an adult congenital disease cohort. Int J Cardiol 2005; 99(2):315–23.

[20] Engel GL. The need for a new medical model: a challenge for biomedicine. Science 1977;196(4286): 129–36.

[21] Moons P, Marquet K, Budts W, et al. Validity, reliability and responsiveness of the "Schedule for the Evaluation of Individual Quality of Life-Direct Weighting" (SEIQoL-DW) in congenital heart disease. Health Qual Life Outcomes 2004;2:27.

[22] Moons P, Van Deyk K, Marquet K, et al. Individual quality of life in adults with congenital heart disease: a paradigm shift. Eur Heart J 2005;26(3):298–307.

[23] Kamphuis M, Ottenkamp J, Vliegen HW, et al. Health related quality of life and health status in adult survivors with previously operated complex congenital heart disease. Heart 2002;87(4):356–62.

[24] Lane DA, Lip GY, Millane TA. Quality of life in adults with congenital heart disease. Heart 2002; 88(1):71–5.

[25] Simko LC, McGinnis KA. Quality of life experienced by adults with congenital heart disease. AACN Clin Issues 2003;14(1):42–53.

[26] Rose M, Kohler K, Kohler F, et al. Determinants of the quality of life of patients with congenital heart disease. Qual Life Res 2005;14(1):35–43.

[27] Gersony WM, Hayes CJ, Driscoll DJ, et al. Second natural history study of congenital heart defects. Quality of life of patients with aortic stenosis, pulmonary stenosis, or ventricular septal defect. Circulation 1993;87(2 Suppl):I52–65.

[28] Saliba Z, Butera G, Bonnet D, et al. Quality of life and perceived health status in surviving adults with univentricular heart. Heart 2001;86(1):69–73.

[29] Immer FF, Althaus SM, Berdat PA, et al. Quality of life and specific problems after cardiac surgery in adolescents and adults with congenital heart diseases. Eur J Cardiovasc Prev Rehabil 2005;12(2):138–43.

[30] Fekkes M, Kamphuis RP, Ottenkamp J, et al. Health-related quality of life in young adults with minor congenital heart disease. Psychol Health 2001;16(2):239–50.

[31] Rietveld S, Mulder BJ, van Beest I, et al. Negative thoughts in adults with congenital heart disease. Int J Cardiol 2002;86(1):19–26.

[32] Simko LC, McGinnis KA. What is the perceived quality of life of adults with congenital heart disease and does it differ by anomaly? J Cardiovasc Nurs 2005;20(3):206–14.

[33] Ternestedt BM, Wall K, Oddsson H, et al. Quality of life 20 and 30 years after surgery in patients operated on for tetralogy of Fallot and for atrial septal defect. Pediatr Cardiol 2001;22(2):128–32.

[34] Moons P, Van Deyk K, De Geest S, et al. Is the severity of congenital heart disease associated with the quality of life and perceived health of adult patients? Heart 2005;91:1193–8.

[35] McMurray R, Kendall L, Parson JM, et al. A life less ordinary: growing up and coping with congenital heart disease. Coron Health Care 2001;5(1):51–7.

[36] Kokkonen J, Paavilainen T. Social adaptation of young adults with congenital heart disease. Int J Cardiol 1992;36(1):23–9.

[37] Tong EM, Sparacino PS, Messias DK, et al. Growing up with congenital heart disease: the dilemmas of adolescents and young adults. Cardiol Young 1998; 8(3):303–9.

[38] Claessens P, Moons P, de Casterle BD, et al. What does it mean to live with a congenital heart disease? A qualitative study on the lived experiences of adult patients. Eur J Cardiovasc Nurs 2005;4(1):3–10.

[39] Kamphuis M, Vogels T, Ottenkamp J, et al. Employment in adults with congenital heart disease. Arch Pediatr Adolesc Med 2002;156(11):1143–8.

[40] Somerville J. The woman with congenital heart disease. Eur Heart J 1998;19(12):1766–75.

[41] Williams RG, Pearson GD, Barst RJ, et al. Report of the National Heart, Lung, and Blood Institute working group on research in adult congenital heart disease. J Am Coll Cardiol 2006;47(4):701–7.

[42] Yusuf S, Hawken S, Ounpuu S, et al, on behalf of the INTERHEART Study Investigators. Effect of potentially modifiable risk factors associated with myocardial infarction in 52 countries (the INTERHEART Study): case-control study. Lancet 2004; 364:937–52.

[43] Rozanski A, Blumenthal JA, Davidson KW, et al. The epidemiology, pathophysiology, and management of psychosocial risk factors in cardiac practice: the emerging field of behavioral cardiology. J Am Coll Cardiol 2005;45(5):637–51.

[44] Zellweger MJ, Osterwalder RH, Langewitz W, et al. Coronary artery disease and depression. Eur Heart J 2004;25(1):3–9.

[45] van Melle JP, de Jonge P, Spijkerman TA, et al. Prognostic association of depression following myocardial infarction with mortality and cardiovascular events: a meta-analysis. Psychosom Med 2004;66(6): 814–22.

[46] Eifert GH, Zvolensky MJ, Lejuez CW. Heart-focused anxiety and chest pain: a conceptual and clinical review. Clin Psychol Sci Prac 2000;7:403–17.

[47] Pauli P, Wiedemann G, Dengler W, et al. Anxiety in patients with an automatic implantable cardioverter

defibrillator: what differentiates them from panic patients? Psychosom Med 1999;61(1):69–76.

[48] Rietveld S, Karsdorp PA, Mulder BJ. Heartbeat sensitivity in adults with congenital heart disease. Int J Behav Med 2004;11(4):203–11.

[49] Price B. Illness careers: the chronic illness experience. J Adv Nurs 1996;24(2):275–9.

[50] Mueller PS, Hook CC, Hayes DL. Ethical analysis of withdrawal of pacemaker or implantable cardioverter-defibrillator support at the end of life. Mayo Clin Proc 2003;78:959–63.

[51] Quill TE, Barold SS, Sussman BL. Discontinuing an implantable cardioverter defibrillator as a life-sustaining treatment. Am J Cardiol 1994;74(2): 205–7.

[52] Kiecolt-Glaser JK, Page GG, Marucha PT, et al. Psychological influences on surgical recovery: perspectives from psychoneuroimmunology. Am Psychol 1998;53(11):1209–18.

[53] Devine EC. Effects of psychoeducational care for adult surgical patients: a meta-analysis of 191 studies. Patient Educ Couns 1992;19(2):129–42.

[54] Johnston M, Vogele C. Benefits of psychological preparation for surgery: a meta-analysis. Ann Beh Med 1993;15:245–56.

[55] Seskevich JE, Crater SW, Lane JD, et al. Beneficial effects of noetic therapies on mood before percutaneous intervention for unstable coronary syndromes. Nurs Res 2004;53(2):116–21.

[56] Gatzoulis K, Frogoudaki A, Brili S, et al. Implantable defibrillators: from the adult cardiac to the grown up congenital heart disease patient. Int J Cardiol 2004;97:117–22.

[57] Herbst JH, Goodman M, Feldstein S, et al. Health related quality of life assessment of patients with life-threatening ventricular arrhythmias. Pacing Clin Electrophysiol 1999;22:915–26.

[58] Schron EB, Exner DV, Yao O, et al. Quality of life in the antiarrhythmics versus implantable defibrillators trial: impact of therapy and influence of adverse symptoms and defibrillator shocks. Circulation 2002;105(5):589–94.

[59] Sears SF, Conti JB. Quality of life and psychological functioning of ICD patients. Heart 2002;87(5): 488–93.

[60] Irvine J, Dorian P, Baker B, et al. Quality of life in the Canadian Implantable Defibrillator Study (CIDS). Am Heart J 2002;144(2):282–9.

[61] Sears SF, Todaro JF, Lewis TS, et al. Examining the psychosocial impact of implantable cardioverter defibrillators: a literature review. Clin Cardiol 1999; 22(7):481–9.

[62] Sears SF, Kovacs AH, Azzarello L, et al. Innovations in health psychology: the psychosocial care of adults with implantable cardioverter defibrillators. Prof Psychol Res Pract 2004;35(5):520–6.

[63] Reid GJ, Irvine MJ, McCrindle BW, et al. Prevalence and correlates of successful transfer from pediatric to adult health care among a cohort of young

adults with complex congenital heart defects. Pediatrics 2004;113:e197–205.

[64] Dusseldorp E, van Elderen T, Maes S, et al. A meta-analysis of psychoeducational programs for coronary heart disease patients. Health Psychol 1999; 18(5):506–19.

[65] Reybrouck T, Mertens L. Physical performance and physical activity in grown-up congenital heart disease. Eur J Cardiovasc Prev Rehabil 2005;12(5): 498–502.

[66] Kulkarni SP, Alexander KP, Lytle B, et al. Long-term adherence with cardiovascular drug regimens. Am Heart J 2006;151(1):185–91.

[67] DiMatteo MR, Lepper HS, Croghan TW. Depression is a risk factor for noncompliance with medical treatment. Meta-analysis of the effects of anxiety and depression on patient adherence. Arch Intern Med 2000;160(14):2102–7.

[68] Ziegelstein RC, Fauerbach JA, Stevens SS, et al. Patients with depression are less likely to follow recommendations to reduce cardiac risk during recovery from a myocardial infarction. Arch Intern Med 2000;160(12):1818–23.

[69] Morgan AL, Masoudi FA, Havranek EP, et al. Difficulty taking medications, depression, and health status in heart failure patients. J Card Fail 2006; 12(1):54–60.

[70] Daliento L, Mapelli D, Volpe B. Measurement of cognitive outcome and quality of life in congenital heart disease. Heart 2006;92(4):569–74.

[71] Bass JL, Corwin M, Gozal D, et al. The effect of chronic or intermittent hypoxia on cognition in childhood: a review of the evidence. Pediatrics 2004;114(3):805–16.

[72] Wray J, Sensky T. Congenital heart disease and cardiac surgery in childhood: effects on cognitive function and academic ability. Heart 2001;85(6):687–91.

[73] Daliento L, Mapelli D, Russo G, et al. Health related quality of life in adults with repaired tetralogy of Fallot: psychosocial and cognitive outcomes. Heart 2005;91:213–8.

[74] Griffin KJ, Elkin TD, Smith CJ. Academic outcomes in children with congenital heart disease. Clin Pediatr 2003;42(5):401–9.

[75] Kamphuis M, Zwinderman KH, Vogels T, et al. A cardiac-specific health related quality of life module for young adults with congenital heart disease: development and validation. Qual Life Res 2004; 13(4):735–45.

[76] Lip GY, Lane DA, Millane TA, et al. Psychological interventions for depression in adolescent and adult congenital heart disease. Cochrane Database Syst Rev 2003;3:CD004394.

[77] Bassett AS, Chow EW, Husted J, et al. Clinical features of 78 adults with 22ql Deletion Syndrome. Am J Med Genet 2005;138A:307–13.

[78] Street RL, Gordon HS, Ward MM, et al. Patient participation in medical consultations: why some patients are more involved than others. Med Care 2005;43(10):960–9.

[79] Salzer MU. Highlights of the meeting of the Psychosocial Working Group of the Association for European Paediatric Cardiology. Cardiol Young 2005; 15(1):111–3.

ELSEVIER
SAUNDERS

Cardiol Clin 24 (2006) 619–629

CARDIOLOGY
CLINICS

# Transition and Transfer from Pediatric to Adult Care of the Young Adult with Complex Congenital Heart Disease

Alison Knauth, MD, PhD[a],*, Amy Verstappen, MEd[b],
John Reiss, PhD[c], Gary D. Webb, MD[d]

[a]Boston Adult Congenital Heart Program, Children's Hospital Boston, Brigham and Women's Hospital, and Harvard
Medical School, 300 Longwood Avenue, Boston, MA 02115, USA
[b]Adult Congenital Heart Association, 6757 Greene Street, Philadelphia, PA 19119, USA
[c]Institute for Child Health Policy, University of Florida, PO Box 100147, Gainesville, FL 32610, USA
[d]Philadelphia Adult Congenital Heart Center, Children's Hospital of Philadelphia and the Hospital of the University
of Pennsylvania, 6 Penn Tower, 3400 Spruce Street, Philadelphia, PA 19104, USA

Many children afflicted with complex childhood illnesses, which historically caused early death, are now surviving childhood with the potential for meaningful and productive adult lives. Although most of these patients eventually transfer their care from a pediatric to an adult health care environment, the process of transitioning, or preparing the patient and family for this transfer, faces many obstacles. As a result transition is neither easy to orchestrate nor simple to perform. An absent or inadequate transition process may result in delayed and inappropriate care, improper timing of the transfer of care, and undue emotional and financial stress for the patients, their families, and the health care system. At its worst, commonly patients are lost to appropriate follow-up. To avoid these hazards, physicians managing these young patients must recognize the importance of the transition process, an educational and experiential process that prepares patients to take responsibility for their own health care. This transition is an important and appropriate process for these young people and marks a significant period in their development as

autonomous patients. It ends by seeing the young patients transfer to an appropriate adult health care setting, one that is better suited to addressing their evolving adult needs and that must continue to do so for the rest of their lives. Performed correctly, the process is challenging but rewarding for these young people and provides them with the opportunity to maximizing their future physical and psychosocial well-being.

This article focuses first on the process of transition (Box 1) and then on the transfer of care for young adults who have chronic childhood illness in general and complex congenital heart disease in specific. It defines the transition process and briefly discusses its history. It then reviews the important aspects of transition, outlines the key elements of a successful transition program, and provides a general curriculum appropriate for the young adult with congenital heart disease. Last, it identifies barriers to the transfer of care, discusses the importance of a policy on the timing of transfer, outlines briefly the components of adult provider services that may be needed, and reviews the steps to an orderly transfer process.

* Corresponding author. Department of Cardiology, Children's Hospital Boston, 300 Longwood Avenue, Boston, MA 02115.
E-mail address: alison.knauth@cardio.chboston.org (A. Knauth).

## Definition of transition and transfer

Transition of care, as referred to in this article, is the process by which adolescents and young adults who have chronic childhood illnesses are

0733-8651/06/$ - see front matter © 2006 Elsevier Inc. All rights reserved.
doi:10.1016/j.ccl.2006.08.010

*cardiology.theclinics.com*

---

**Box 1. Key elements of a transition
and transfer program**

- Development of program for patient
  preparation and education
  - Well-structured curriculum
  - Choice of multiple educational
    modalities
    - Clinic visits
    - Educational seminars
    - Peer support groups

- Identification of obstacles to transfer of
  care
  - Patients
  - Families
  - Pediatric caregivers
  - Adult caregivers

- Establishment of (flexible) policy on
  timing of transfer

- Identification of capable and available
  adult providers

- Plan for a coordinated transfer
  - Coordinator
  - Written health summary
  - Direct communications between
    caregivers

---

prepared to take charge of their lives and their health in adulthood. It is an educational process that ideally begins before children reach adolescence and continues until they are capable of taking full responsibility for their care. Most importantly, young patients who have complex congenital heart disease are taught that, although they have the potential to live healthy and productive lives, they have been "repaired" and not "cured"; they require lifelong cardiac surveillance, and they are responsible for obtaining appropriate care.

Transfer defines an event or series of events through which adolescents and young adults who have chronic physical and medical conditions move their care from a pediatric to an adult health care environment. It is important that transfer be deferred in the absence of appropriate adult resources. If appropriate adult care is available, however, transfer is likely to be beneficial to patients. Although a pediatric care model is ideal for young children, as it focuses on growth and

development and directs education toward the parents or guardians, it is no longer appropriate for adult patients. The adult care model, in contrast, employs a visit dynamic that is a more of a partnership with education directed toward the patients, thus encouraging independence, responsibility, and self-reliance. The goal is a smooth transfer following a structured transition program provided by pediatric and adolescent providers.

## A brief history of transition

Health care transition for young people who have chronic health conditions has long been recommended [1–3]. In the United States, multiple invitational conferences and task forces have identified the problems faced by the growing population of adults who had chronic childhood illnesses and their need for formal transition programs. In 2003, the American Academy of Pediatrics, American Academy of Family Physicians, and American College of Physicians presented a consensus statement on health care transition for young adults who have special health care needs [4]. This statement was endorsed by the Society for Adolescent Medicine in its 2003 position paper [5]. Similarly, in the United Kingdom, the transition of young adults who have chronic childhood illnesses to the adult health care system was addressed explicitly by the Royal College of Pediatrics and Child Health in recently released guidelines on health care for adolescents [6].

Specialty professional organizations also have weighed in on the need for transition programs with editorials, practice guidelines, and position statements related to the transition of young people who have specific health concerns. In particular, the needs of adults who have congenital heart disease and recommendations for transition and transfer of care have been formalized by a number of expert task forces including the 32nd Bethesda Conference convened by the American College of Cardiology [7–11], the Canadian Cardiovascular Society Consensus Conference [12–14], and the British Cardiac Society [6,15]. Perhaps even more compelling is that patients, most notably the Adult Congenital Heart Association, are asking for transition programs by organizing work groups to address these issues and to promote the formation of programs across the country.

Despite the recognized need for transition programs, most adolescent patients still do not have the opportunity to participate in such a process. It is hoped that this situation will change as the endorsement of health care transition grows, broader ranges of transition experience are described, and steps are taken to evaluate such programs formally [16–22].

## Goals of the transition process

Few would argue with the appropriateness of and benefits associated with preparing young people to take charge of their own health and lives. Nevertheless, the smooth transition to this state remains a challenge for everyone involved. With this challenge in mind, formal structured transition programs have been proposed [5,6,22–24]. The goals of such programs are several. First and foremost, they aim to provide uninterrupted health care that is patient centered, age and developmentally appropriate, flexible, and comprehensive. Young people are coached to make a smooth transfer from a pediatric to an adult health care environment without becoming lost to follow-up. Transition programs are committed to educating young people about their medical conditions and promoting skills in communication, decision making, self-care, and self-advocacy. As a result, patients become capable of personal and medical independence and gain a greater sense of control over their health, health care decisions, and psychosocial environment. The ultimate goal of transition programs is to optimize the quality of life and future potential of young patients [2].

## Transition needs of adults who have congenital heart disease

Adolescents who have congenital heart disease constitute a growing population of individuals who have such complex medical issues that a well-planned and well-executed transition process can be valuable. Because of advances in pediatric cardiovascular surgery, percutaneous interventional therapies, intensive care, and medical management, many children who have complex congenital heart disease are now surviving into adulthood. As a result, the number of adults who have congenital heart disease in the United States is rising steadily and currently nears 1 million. Half of these patients have complex congenital heart conditions for which most adult cardiologists have not been trained. In addition, they often present with complex comorbidities and psychosocial challenges. These patients need lifelong care

by specialized practitioners who are fluent in the complex anatomy and physiology of congenital heart disease and who are well versed in the lexis of adult internal medicine [7–11,25].

## Models of transition

A variety of transition models have been proposed, including generic and disease-based models, and transition recommendations have been elaborated and published. The generic transition model employs adolescent medicine services to run generic transition programs designed to address general adolescent and transition issues while relying on subspecialty programs to handle specific medical issues. The disease-based model carries out the transition process within a program that specializes in the medical needs of a particular type of childhood illness. This model has the benefit of being able to tailor the transition process to the individual patient [23,26]. The disease-based model may be best for young adults who have congenital heart disease, given the heterogeneity of the population and the complexity of their medical conditions. In the absence of such a program, much of the responsibility for transition falls on pediatric providers using a less formal approach.

## Key elements of transition

Regardless of the model, fundamental principles of transition have achieved nearly universal endorsement [6,19,23]. These principles provide a framework for individual programs and institutions whose goal is to improve the transition experience for their young adult patients who have chronic health conditions. The following discussion outlines what the authors believe are the key elements that must be incorporated into a transition program. These key elements begin with patient preparation and education using a well-structured curriculum, require the recognition of the obstacles to transition and transfer that must be proactively addressed, and depend on a policy regarding the timing of transfer, the identification of appropriate adult provider services, and a coordinated transfer process.

### Preparation and education

Although a formal transition curriculum is most appropriate during late childhood and adolescence, preparation for successful transition should begin early and continue throughout childhood. A major potential barrier to successful transition is the mistaken perception of families and patients that a "cure" has resulted from successful cardiac surgery. Such misperceptions should be solicited regularly and addressed directly. Patients and families must understand that, although in many cases their children are likely to have a normal or near-normal life, they do not have a normal heart and will require lifelong surveillance. Furthermore, they must be taught that congenital heart disease is vastly different from other forms of heart disease, making it imperative that they follow up with providers specializing in adult congenital heart disease. From early in the course of care, families should have the expectation that their children will be independent in managing their own medical care by young adulthood. Families should be encouraged to help their children reach this goal. Providers must help families build their children's knowledge of their heart disease using age-appropriate strategies [23,27,28]. Core concepts should be revisited regularly, because medical concepts are complex, and educational research has shown that repetition greatly enhances retention and understanding [29]. Ideally, using such a strategy of early preparation, the patients and families will enter the transition period with an understanding of their heart disease and the need for lifelong specialized care.

Building on this preparation, the transition curriculum should ensure that these young people understand their diagnosis and medical history. Ideally, they must understand the normal heart (basic anatomy and physiology), how the heart they were born with differs from normal, and what surgical or catheter-based interventions were undertaken to "repair" their heart. Because these young people already understand that "repair" does not mean "cure," they will be ready to learn about the risks of residual hemodynamic burdens and arrhythmic complications. They should be taught to recognize important signs and symptoms that may alert them to such complications. The transitioning adolescents should have a good understanding of the rationale for previous therapies and options for future medical, surgical, and catheter-based therapies. Finally, they need to be prepared to navigate the adult health care system: how to access an adult congenital heart specialist, how often they need such follow-up, how to access routine health care, how to access emergency health care, and how to navigate the insurance process.

*The transition curriculum*

A standard core educational program (Box 2) is an important component of an organized transition process. The goals of this curriculum can be achieved using a variety of educational modalities and should be tailored to individual patients. The curriculum should be of appropriate breadth and depth but concise enough to be completed before patients move into the adult congenital heart disease clinic. Completion of the curriculum may require two clinic visits for mature, well-adjusted patients who have mild disease, mild functional limitations, and a strong support system or many visits with intense involvement of a peer support group for a young person who has learning disabilities, complex disease, significant functional limitations, and no support system. Flexibility is a key to success.

The elements of a transition curriculum include both medical and nonmedical issues and are outlined below. The curriculum goals can be accomplished in a number of different ways. Much of the curriculum can be addressed at routinely scheduled clinic visits with the participation of physicians, midlevel practitioners, and support services. Additionally, a transition program can design introductory seminars for patients and families or use peer support groups and informational seminars to address some of the components of the transition curriculum.

*Residual hemodynamic considerations*

Most patients who have repaired congenital heart disease have residual hemodynamic burdens. Honest discussions are required regarding these residual hemodynamic issues, their implications for the future, and the signs and symptoms that should raise concern. Patients should be told about future diagnostic testing required to keep these matters under appropriate surveillance. In addition, they should be educated about the possible medical, catheter-based, or surgical options for treating these problems if or when they are needed.

It also is important to discuss new advances in cardiovascular medicine including advances in medical management, cardiac catheterization, and cardiovascular surgery. Such discussions often can be accomplished effectively in peer support groups and informational seminars. Through this education, young people can develop a positive and hopeful outlook for the future despite the knowledge of potential future

**Box 2. Transition curriculum topics**

- Residual hemodynamic considerations
  - Hemodynamic issues
  - Symptoms and how to respond
  - Diagnostic tools in follow-up
  - Management options

- Contraception and pregnancy planning
  - Contraceptive options and risks
  - Risks of pregnancy to mother and to fetus
  - Management of pregnancy plan

- Endocarditis considerations
  - Risks, implications, recognition, and response
  - Prevention

- Arrhythmia considerations
  - Risks
  - Signs and symptoms
  - Screening tools
  - Diagnostic tools
  - Management options

- Noncardiac surgery considerations
  - Risks
  - Location of surgery
  - Knowledge and skills of surgical and ICU team

- Noncardiac medical problems
  - Access to appropriate care

- Career and vocational planning

- Lifestyle issues
  - Marriage and family planning
  - Education
  - Employment
  - Life and health insurance
  - Learning disabilities
  - Anxiety and depression
  - High-risk behaviors
  - Healthy eating
  - Physical fitness
  - Salt and fluid restriction (if warranted)
  - Relative safety of exercise and hobbies

- End-of-life decisions

- Skills training

- Communication
- Decision making
- Creative problem solving
- Assertiveness
- Self-care
- Self-advocacy

complications. Giving patients tools to learn about such therapies on their own and encouraging them to seek new knowledge continuously enables them to feel a sense of control over their health and medical management.

*Contraception and pregnancy planning*

It is important that discussions about contraception and pregnancy occur before patients reach adolescence. It is common for young people to transfer abruptly to the adult health care system as a result of an unplanned pregnancy. Pregnancy, especially in a woman who has complex congenital heart disease, should be well planned to minimize risks to the mother and unborn child. The young person should have the opportunity to make an informed decision about if and when to become pregnant. For this reason, contraceptive options should be discussed with patients before they become sexually active. During these conversations, it must be emphasized that the various contraceptive options carry both benefits and risks. For example, estrogen-containing oral contraceptive pills increase the risk of thromboembolism and may not be recommended in certain patients. Beyond pregnancy planning or prevention, information about barrier methods for prevention of sexually transmitted diseases always should be provided.

Pregnancy *is* feasible for many adult patients who have congenital heart disease, but the potential risks to the mother and unborn child should be discussed before conception. Frank discussions should be had regarding the severity of the patients, underlying disease and relative risk of complications during pregnancy, delivery, and postpartum, as well as possible risks to the fetus such as poor growth, premature labor and delivery, and the chance of congenital heart disease. Fetal echocardiography and genetic counseling should be offered in selected cases. Finally, the development of a realistic plan regarding the timing of and most appropriate number of pregnancies may be desirable.

## Endocarditis considerations

Few adolescents who have congenital heart disease understand what endocarditis is and why they are more likely than the general population to suffer this complication [27]. As a standard part of a transition curriculum, patients should be educated about the implications of endocarditis. They should learn how to reduce the risk of endocarditis through attention to oral health and the use appropriate antibiotic prophylaxis. Finally, they should be able to recognize the signs and symptoms of endovascular infection so they know to seek medical attention promptly.

## Arrhythmia considerations

Arrhythmias are a relatively common complication experienced by patients who have congenital heart disease, and patients should be educated about them when relevant. It is important that patients understand what atrial and ventricular arrhythmias are, their causation, and the relative risk or hazard of each (tailored to each individual patient). An explanation and understanding of which arrhythmias are simply an annoyance, which may be life threatening, and how to recognize the signs and symptoms that should raise concern are necessary. Patients should understand the importance of screening tools and the potential need for other diagnostic tests if concerning signs or symptoms arise. Finally, arrhythmia management, including medications, radiofrequency catheter ablation, surgical ablation, and device therapies (pacemakers and defibrillators), should be discussed as needed.

## Noncardiac surgery considerations

Patients need to be advised about the issues regarding noncardiac surgery. Important considerations include the need for the treating team to be informed fully about the patients, heart condition. Except for the simplest outpatient procedures, noncardiac surgeries in complex patients should be performed in a tertiary hospital where cardiac anesthesiologists, as well as other members of the surgical and critical care teams, are comfortable with the care of adults who have congenital heart disease. Knowledge about these issues allows patients to serve as their own advocates.

## Noncardiac medical problems

Discussions about noncardiac medical problems must be tailored to the individual patient. Patients should be aware of the implications of these issues and know how to access appropriate care.

## Career, vocational, and insurance planning

Many adolescents who have congenital heart disease will be able to plan their education and careers in a normal fashion. The futures of some will include physical or other limitations, however, and they should be advised to pursue education and careers that are sustainable even if physical limitations develop. It is important that this part of the process begin before patients reach high school, when they will make academic choices that can limit future options. In addition, it is important to teach these young patients that adults who have complex congenital heart disease are likely to have difficulties securing health insurance independently, and therefore obtaining a health plan through an employer may be optimal. Life insurance poses similar obstacles, and often early and disciplined self-investment is desirable.

## Lifestyle issues

Because the goal of all medical care is to improve the quality of life for the patient, a transition curriculum must at some point depart from the medical realm and include discussions about lifestyle and quality of life. These include marriage and family planning, education, employment, and life and health insurance. Other challenges faced by young people who have congenital heart disease, such as learning disabilities, anxiety and depression, and high-risk behaviors, including use of tobacco, alcohol, and other drugs of abuse, should be acknowledged. It is important that these discussions be held in private, in a safe and comfortable environment. The importance of healthful eating and physical fitness, the risks of poor nutrition and obesity, and the need for salt and fluid restriction (if warranted) should be addressed. Education regarding appropriate diet and exercise can be accomplished effectively in informational seminars and peer support groups. Finally, the relative safety of exercise and other hobbies should be discussed.

## End-of-life decisions

Anyone may have to make end-of-life decisions. Young people who have chronic childhood illnesses may face these decisions sooner than their healthy peers. It is well known that these decisions are made most effectively during a time of health rather than urgently at a time of acute illness or worsening chronic disease. For this reason discussions about these decisions should be included in the transition process. In addition, informational seminars and peer support groups may be effective ways for young people to discuss their ideas, fears, and plans.

*Skills training*

The transition program curriculum should include skills training in communication, decision making, creative problem solving, assertiveness, self-care, self-determination, and self-advocacy. Much of this training can be accomplished in informational seminars and peer support groups and reinforced at clinic visits.

## Obstacles to transfer of care

Although many barriers exist to the successful transfer of congenital heart patients out of pediatric cardiac care, only a few young adults who have complex congenital heart problems continue to receive care from their pediatric cardiologists. Currently, the majority of adults who have congenital heart disease experience unplanned transfer without transition; they discontinue care with their pediatric team at some point in adolescence or young adulthood and later transfer to an adult health care environment without preparation, education, or a plan. Research suggests that the majority of adults who have complex congenital heart disease are either lost from cardiac care entirely or are cared for by cardiologists without specialized training [30,31].

For patients still being seen in the pediatric care system, there are many obstacles to a smooth transfer process, both intrinsic and extrinsic to the physician–patient team, and a successful transfer must address these issues [1,23,32]. Obstacles that lie outside the patient–physician relationship are often the most obvious. These obstacles include problems accessing competent adult care that can match the quality of care and range of services available in the pediatric environment as well as financial and insurance issues.

Less obvious, and often more difficult to address, are obstacles that lie within the physician–patient axis. First, the adolescents themselves may impede their own progress. Transferring care may be traumatic for the young person. The challenge of accepting their new

responsibility for their own health and lives can be overwhelming, and adolescents may subconsciously see the transfer of care as a danger rather than an opportunity. Moreover, at this time of personal adolescent struggle, they are forced to give up their relationships with trusted and respected pediatric care providers and are expected to develop new relationships with an unknown group. They may be expected to transfer from a pediatric facility within which they feel comfortable to an adult facility that is anything but coddling. Finally, the self-image of young people who have chronic illness is often infantilized, promoting dependence. The transfer of care to the adult health care system challenges patients to become independent and may be resisted.

Similarly, patients' families can be unwitting obstacles to the transfer of their children's care. Adult care models usually take an individual approach rather than a family approach, and although this approach encourages patient autonomy and self-dependence, the families of these patients often feel excluded from this new dynamic. Some parents perceive this difference in approach as a loss of control and thus resist any change in the status quo, rather than viewing transfer as a positive step toward greater autonomy and self-sufficiency for their maturing adolescent. In addition, families are often concerned that their children will not be capable of caring for their illness independently, further contributing to resistance to the transfer. Finally, like their adolescent children, families are reluctant to change from the known and trusted pediatric providers and facilities to the unknown adult system. They often are concerned that the care will be impersonal or less skilled. For these reasons, a successful transition program must explicitly acknowledge and address the expected shift in family dynamics and be prepared to assist and counsel families who have particular difficulty in stepping back and letting go of their previous intimate role in their children's care. It must be emphasized to the families that the transfer of care is ultimately a positive step for their children toward reaching their full potential.

The pediatric provider also can be an obstacle to the transition process. Too often the provider is unable to relinquish the intense and important relationship that has developed with these patients and families. The impact that the loss of such relationships imposes on the pediatric providers is often underestimated. In addition, pediatric providers may be skeptical about the knowledge, skills, and experience of the adult providers and may communicate this attitude to their young patients in explicit or implicit ways, making them wary of transfer. The point should be emphasized again: important though transfer may be, it always should be to competent adult care. It would be unacceptable to put patients at risk by transferring their care to unskilled providers.

Finally, the adult service may pose a significant obstacle. Adult providers may be intimidated by the complexity of these patients and may recognize the care of these patients as a financial liability. When willing to take on such complex patients, adult providers may wish to embark on an extensive reevaluation or a prompt change in management, which can be unsettling to patients and families. The transfer of medical records and communication between pediatric and adult providers is not always well done and can compound these problems. Anticipation and avoidance of these obstacles to transfer is preferable to struggling with them as they arise.

### The timing of transfer

Ideally, transfer of care from a pediatric to an adult health care system occurs at the successful completion of a thoughtful transition process. When deciding on the timing of transfer, two important points need to be considered. First, there should be a policy on timing to ensure that transition and transfer actually occur and occur in a predictable manner [23]. Second, despite the policy on timing, a transition program must be flexible and should tailor the transfer process and its timing to the developmental and psychosocial status of each young person [26,32].

Each institution requires a policy on the age at which its patients will transfer to appropriate adult care. It is important for care providers, patients, and families to have an explicit target age. With such a policy, patients and families recognize that transition and transfer will occur, appreciate their active involvement in the decisions about timing, and are prepared for the ultimate transfer of care. Additionally, when transition is the rule, young people see the process not as something they as individuals are forced to go through alone but rather a natural process that everyone experiences: much as high school follows junior high school, so adult care follows pediatric care. Finally, a policy on timing ensures that everyone involved in the process has the time and

opportunity to take full advantage of the entire transition curriculum.

Uncompromising structure frequently is only marginally better than chaos, and neither has a place in a well-organized transition process. It therefore is important to remember that the presence of structure in this process should never preclude rational plasticity—the timing of transfer must be flexible. Important decisions about timing must be individualized to each young person and should occur in a developmental context. Transitioning should be introduced early, as previously emphasized, and should be completed only after the young patients have accomplished the developmental tasks of adolescence and have demonstrated the ability to manage their health care independently of their families and pediatric providers.

Early introduction of the concepts of transition and transfer to patients and their families is critical [16,17] and should occur before the child enters the developmental stage of adolescence. At the initiation of these discussions, it may be helpful for the patients and families to write an individualized transition plan that includes a timeline. This written document can be reviewed and revised at intervals. In this way, the patients and families participate actively in the transition process and are aware and prepared for the ultimate transfer of care.

Adolescents have many difficult tasks to accomplish before leaving this stage in their development, namely, to develop a personal sense of identity and adjust to this new physical sense of self; to adjust to new intellectual abilities and the increased cognitive demands placed on them at school and in society in general; to develop educational and vocational goals for themselves and a plan to meet these goals; to establish emotional and psychologic independence from their parents and begin to adopt a personal value system; to learn to manage their sexuality and begin to develop intimate relationships; and to develop increased impulse control and behavioral maturity. Chronic illness, physical disability, and cognitive limitations can disrupt the usual developmental trajectories. This interruption makes the accomplishment of such tasks more difficult, and thus the process of transition may be more challenging [24,26].

Furthermore, the sometimes overprotective attitudes of pediatric providers and patients' families can diminish self-esteem and hinder the development of self-sufficiency. In general, the adult health care system demands a higher level of personal responsibility and autonomy than the pediatric system. Thus, to be effective health care consumers in the adult health care environment, young people should demonstrate the ability to meet their health care needs independently of their families and pediatric providers before transfer. They need to have the ability to make their own appointments, meet independently with their health care providers, administer their own medications and other treatments, understand their medical history, and recognize signs of clinical deterioration.

Finally, transfer of care during medical crises or periods of psychosocial disequilibrium should be avoided [23]. All too often patients are transferred when they become pregnant or after they suffer their first "adult" complication. Transfer during these times precludes maximal use of the transition curriculum and imposes a tremendous psychologic burden on the existing crisis. A structured policy on timing of transfer helps ensure that the process is begun before many of these crises have the opportunity to develop and the flexibility to defer transfer until acute issues are addressed; thus a structured policy reduces the psychosocial burden for patients.

**Adult provider services**

Although the needs of some patients are relatively straightforward, other patients have complex needs and may require the involvement of a variety of consultants, including an electrophysiologist, psychiatrist, obstetrician, gynecologist, gastroenterologist, hepatologist, nephrologist, pulmonologist, neurologist, or oncologist. Other medical and nonmedical professionals, including midlevel providers, social workers, and those who specialize in vocational and educational issues, are also critical to successful transition [8,10,23].

In addition, young people who have chronic health conditions require capable primary health care providers willing to coordinate and manage the complex care they need [6]. Young people who have chronic conditions share many of the same health issues and concerns as their peers, namely, growth and development; sexuality; depression and other mental health disorders; substance use; and other high-risk behaviors. The primary care providers who take on this population of patients must be prepared to address these issues themselves or to ensure they are being addressed in other settings. The specialist often will not address other medical issues; thus the role of primary care providers should be defined explicitly. Communication between specialists and primary care providers is paramount.

**Coordinated transfer process**

A coordinated transfer process is the final component of a successful transition process [17,22,23]. As the time for transfer approaches, preparations need to be made to ensure the process goes smoothly. By now, the patients and their families have been prepared through the transition program and are ready for the transfer of care. A carefully prepared health summary allows seamless transfer of care and provides a blueprint for the new health care team, especially early after transfer. A comprehensive summary should include a complete medical history including diagnoses and previous interventions, a medication list, laboratory values, and other diagnostic studies, as well as information about the patient's functional status, the tempo of disease progression, and the impact of other comorbidities. Psychosocial concerns, end-of-life preferences, the extent of family involvement, and adherence issues should also be communicated if available. A comprehensive summary avoids the need to reinvent the therapeutic wheel and helps prevent errors being made or mistakes being repeated. In addition to the formal medical summary, it is vital that the pediatric providers, including the specialist physicians, physical and occupational therapists, dietitians, social workers, nurses, and other health-care professionals, communicate directly with their counterparts in the adult health care system.

It is important that the adult providers respect the therapeutic plan established by the pediatric providers and communicated to the young patients and their families. As explained earlier, the immediate reevaluation and drastic change in management that many new adult providers are tempted to make after care transfer often can be overwhelming to the patients and diminish their trust. Nonetheless, one must also take advantage of the unique opportunity this transition process provides to take a fresh look at the patients as evolving adults and to reassess therapeutic options in the light of new technologies. This process can be done in conjunction with the pediatric providers and after a period of introduction and relationship development in the transition process. In this way trust is not lost, and the best possible plan for the future is made.

Many transition tools have been suggested to aid in a smooth transition process. For example, a central care provider who can assume responsibility for progress through the process of transition and transfer has been shown to be helpful [17,22]. This coordinator can share membership on both the pediatric and adult teams and serve as a liaison between them, as well as a reassuring presence and advocate for families. In addition, there are a number of ways to help address the inevitable uncertainty felt by young people and their families about impending transfer. Many programs have created a transfer package with information and details about the adult program, including its providers and procedures [17]. Patients who have already transferred to the adult program sometimes can play a part in welcoming young people who are newly transferring their care.

## Summary

Because increasing numbers of young people who have complex congenital illnesses are surviving into adulthood, there is an urgent need for programs designed to facilitate their smooth movement from pediatric to adult health care environments. This article has identified the important constituents of the transition process and has provided guidelines to the successful transfer of the patient to the adult health care environment. In the near future, it is hoped, transition programs will become the standard of care, making it more likely that patients who have complex congenital heart disease can achieve their full potential under appropriate medical surveillance and live meaningful and productive lives.

## References

[1] Schidlow DV, Fiel SB. Life beyond pediatrics. Transition of chronically ill adolescents from pediatric to adult health care systems. Med Clin North Am 1990; 74(5):1113–20.

[2] Blum RW, Garell D, Hodgman CH, et al. Transition from child-centered to adult health-care systems for adolescents with chronic conditions. A position paper of the Society for Adolescent Medicine. J Adolesc Health 1993;14(7):570–6.

[3] Rosen DS. Transition from pediatric to adult-oriented health care for the adolescent with chronic illness or disability. Adolesc Med 1994; 5(2):241–8.

[4] A consensus statement on health care transitions for young adults with special health care needs. Pediatrics 2002;110(6 Pt 2):1304–6.

[5] Rosen DS, Blum RW, Britto M, et al. Transition to adult health care for adolescents and young adults with chronic conditions: position paper of the Society for Adolescent Medicine. J Adolesc Health 2003;33(4):309–11.

[6] Grown-up congenital heart (GUCH) disease: current needs and provision of service for adolescents and adults with congenital heart disease in the UK. Heart 2002;88(Suppl 1):i1–14.

[7] Warnes CA, Liberthson R, Danielson GK, et al. Task force 1: the changing profile of congenital heart disease in adult life. J Am Coll Cardiol 2001;37(5): 1170–5.

[8] Foster E, Graham TP Jr, Driscoll DJ, et al. Task force 2: special health care needs of adults with congenital heart disease. J Am Coll Cardiol 2001;37(5): 1176–83.

[9] Child JS, Collins-Nakai RL, Alpert JS, et al. Task force 3: workforce description and educational requirements for the care of adults with congenital heart disease. J Am Coll Cardiol 2001;37(5):1183–7.

[10] Landzberg MJ, Murphy DJ Jr, Davidson WR Jr, et al. Task force 4: organization of delivery systems for adults with congenital heart disease. J Am Coll Cardiol 2001;37(5):1187–93.

[11] Skorton DJ, Garson A Jr, Allen HD, et al. Task force 5: adults with congenital heart disease: access to care. J Am Coll Cardiol 2001;37(5): 1193–8.

[12] Therrien J, Dore A, Gersony W, et al. Canadian Cardiovascular Society consensus conference 2001 update: recommendations for the management of adults with congenital heart disease. Part I. Can J Cardiol 2001;17(9):940–59.

[13] Therrien J, Gatzoulis M, Graham T, et al. Canadian Cardiovascular Society consensus conference 2001 update: recommendations for the management of adults with congenital heart disease—part II. Can J Cardiol 2001;17(10):1029–50.

[14] Therrien J, Warnes C, Daliento L, et al. Canadian Cardiovascular Society consensus conference 2001 update: recommendations for the management of adults with congenital heart disease: part III. Can J Cardiol 2001;17(11):1135–58.

[15] British Cardiac Society and the Royal College of Physicians of London. The future of paediatric cardiology in the United Kingdom. Br Heart J 1992; 68(6):630–3.

[16] Boyle MP, Farukhi Z, Nosky ML. Strategies for improving transition to adult cystic fibrosis care, based on patient and parent views. Pediatr Pulmonol 2001; 32(6):428–36.

[17] Madge S, Bryon M. A model for transition from pediatric to adult care in cystic fibrosis. J Pediatr Nurs 2002;17(4):283–8.

[18] Kipps S, Bahu T, Ong K, et al. Current methods of transfer of young people with Type 1 diabetes to adult services. Diabet Med 2002;19(8):649–54.

[19] Fernandes SM, Landzberg MJ. Transitioning the young adult with congenital heart disease for lifelong medical care. Pediatr Clin North Am 2004; 51(6):1739–48 [xi.].

[20] Reid GJ, Irvine MJ, McCrindle BW, et al. Prevalence and correlates of successful transfer from pediatric to adult health care among a cohort of young adults with complex congenital heart defects. Pediatrics 2004;113(3 Pt 1):e197–205.

[21] Williams WG, McCrindle BW. Practical experience with databases for congenital heart disease: a registry versus an academic database. Semin Thorac Cardiovasc Surg Pediatr Card Surg Annu 2002;5:132–42.

[22] Viner R. Barriers and good practice in transition from paediatric to adult care. J R Soc Med 2001; 94(Suppl 40):2–4.

[23] Viner R. Bridging the gaps: transition for young people with cancer. Eur J Cancer 2003;39(18):2684–7.

[24] Hergenroeder AC. The transition into adulthood for children and youth with special health care needs. Tex Med 2002;98(2):51–8.

[25] Murphy DJ Jr, Foster E. ACCF/AHA/AAP recommendations for training in pediatric cardiology. Task force 6: training in transition of adolescent care and care of the adult with congenital heart disease. J Am Coll Cardiol 2005;46(7):1399–401.

[26] Bryon M, Madge S. Transition from paediatric to adult care: psychological principles. J R Soc Med 2001;94(Suppl 40):5–7.

[27] Moons P, De Volder E, Budts W, et al. What do adult patients with congenital heart disease know about their disease, treatment, and prevention of complications? A call for structured patient education. Heart 2001;86(1):74–80.

[28] Webb GD. Challenges in the care of adult patients with congenital heart defects. Heart 2003;89(4): 465–9.

[29] Bransford JDBA, Cocking RR. How people learn: brain, mind, experience, and school. Committee on Developments in the Science of Learning, Commission on Behavioral and Social Sciences and Education, National Research Council. Washington (DC): National Academy Press; 1999. p. 39–67.

[30] Dore A, de Guise P, Mercier LA. Transition of care to adult congenital heart centres: what do patients know about their heart condition? Can J Cardiol 2002;18(2):141–6.

[31] Wacker A, Kaemmerer H, Hollweck R, et al. Outcome of operated and unoperated adults with congenital cardiac disease lost to follow-up for more than five years. Am J Cardiol 2005; 95(6):776–9.

[32] Rosen D. Between two worlds: bridging the cultures of child health and adult medicine. J Adolesc Health 1995;17(1):10–6.

CARDIOLOGY
CLINICS

Cardiol Clin 24 (2006) 631–639

# Determinants and Assessment of Pulmonary Regurgitation in Tetralogy of Fallot: Practice and Pitfalls

Andrew N. Redington, MD

*Division of Cardiology, Hospital for Sick Children, 555 University Avenue, Toronto, Ontario M5G 1X8, Canada*

During the last two decades, a remarkable turnaround has occurred in understanding the effects of pulmonary regurgitation after the repair of tetralogy of Fallot. Previously thought to be a benign consequence of outflow tract surgery, it is now recognized as the single most important determinant of late outcome. Indeed, deterioration in right ventricular function, exercise performance, and the propensity to ventricular arrhythmia can all be traced back to the secondary effects of pulmonary regurgitation.

The goal of this article is not to describe the secondary effects but rather the primary determinants of pulmonary regurgitation. Furthermore, the methods by which pulmonary regurgitation is measured and some of the pitfalls therein are highlighted.

## Determinants of pulmonary regurgitation

There are four determinants of semilunar valve regurgitation (Fig. 1): (1) the size of the regurgitant orifice, (2) the hydraulic impedance/afterload, (3) the ventricular diastolic compliance, and (4) the diastolic filling time. In aortic regurgitation, the difference between hydraulic impedance/afterload and ventricular compliance is an overwhelming and relatively fixed determinant of regurgitant flow; however, because of the low pressure, low impedance nature of the pulmonary vascular bed, a "freely" regurgitant outflow tract can be tolerated for decades. Nonetheless, relatively subtle changes

in these variables can lead to a major change in the absolute volume of pulmonary incompetence. For a full understanding of the amount of pulmonary incompetence in a given patient, each of these variables must be taken into account.

### Regurgitant valve orifice

The normal right ventricular outflow tract is a complex structure [1]. The pulmonary valve is a free-standing structure separate from the fibrous skeleton of the heart that provides a supporting superstructure to the tricuspid, mitral, and aortic valves. Sitting on a complete muscular infundibulum, the integrity of the pulmonary valve leaflets themselves will vary not only with the integrity of the valve but also with the dynamic nature of the muscular infundibulum and the size of the immediate supravalve area. Gross right heart dilatation, regardless of the cause, can lead to important pulmonary regurgitation as the muscular outflow tract dilates. There is no anatomic fibrous ring supporting the pulmonary valve leaflets; rather, there is a muscular to fibrous connection at the point of the ventriculoarterial junction. The pulmonary valve leaflets are arranged in semilunar fashion, traversing the muscular and fibrous elements, as in the aortic valve [1]. Thus, it is easy to imagine that supravalve or subvalve dilatation (iatrogenic or secondary) could undermine the function of the semilunar valve leaflets, even if their integrity was preserved at the time of repair.

Rarely does a patient with tetralogy of Fallot not require enlargement of the outflow tract in some way (beyond resection of the outlet septum); therefore, surgery to the sinuses and supravalve

*E-mail address:* andrew.redington@sickkids.ca

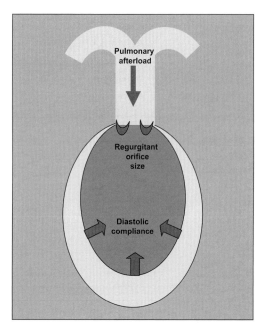

Fig. 1. Schematic demonstrating the determinants of pulmonary regurgitation. The pulmonary artery afterload, regurgitant orifice, and diastolic compliance of the right ventricle are all independent variables in individual patients.

area, enlargement of the ventriculoarterial junction, enlargement of the subpulmonary infundibulum, or a combination of one or more procedures in the form of a transannular patch are variable elements of the repair. Perhaps because of a lack of understanding of the late sequelae of pulmonary regurgitation and the early reports of the adverse effects of residual stenosis at the time of primary repair [2], surgeons have erred on the side of "complete" relief of stenosis at the expense of regurgitation. Indeed, resection of pulmonary valve leaflets in association with the transannular patch was de rigueur in the 1960s and 1970s. Subsequently, there has been an increasing trend toward preservation of the pulmonary outflow tract at the time of primary repair.

The paranoia regarding residual outflow tract obstruction seems to be less relevant in the contemporary era. Surgical mortality is extremely low as is interval mortality in the first years after surgery, despite degrees of residual stenosis considered intolerable in previous eras. It also recognized that the diminutive outflow tract may grow, even if residual stenosis remains at the end of the primary procedure. Antunes and coworkers [3] showed clearly that residual pressure gradients generally

fell over the first 12 months after surgery in a series in which transannular patches were avoided in the vast majority of patients. More recently, the Toronto group has demonstrated the early benefits and the high rate of success with valve-sparing procedures [4]. Over 70% of unselected patients were able to avoid transannular patches when a protocol including deferred repair to the age of 3 to 6 months was instituted. Modest residual gradients tended not to progress, and many regressed during the first years after surgery. There was a small risk for the need of reoperation. Nevertheless, there is an increasing trend toward early primary repair at the time of diagnosis in the neonatal period. Although this procedure can now be performed with an extremely low mortality, the consequence of this approach is a much higher transannular patch rate, often greater than 70% [5]. It remains to be seen whether the combination of early surgical repair, with its stated aim of preserving right ventricular diastolic function, in combination with a transannular patch might lead to more long-term problems than more conservative approaches. This is a complex question because, for the reasons outlined previously, even the more conservative approaches, such as isolated outflow tract and supra-annular patching, may ultimately provide the substrate for free pulmonary regurgitation.

One should remember that even the circumstances of free pulmonary incompetence do not equate directly to "severe" pulmonary incompetence. This extremely important concept ties into the nature of semilunar valve regurgitation. The volume of regurgitation will vary markedly, even across a potentially freely regurgitant valve orifice, depending on the balance of afterload in the pulmonary vascular bed and right ventricular diastolic function.

*Pulmonary vascular bed*

It has long been known anecdotally that the combination of a transannular patch and distal pulmonary artery stenosis is a particularly malignant combination in terms of the evolution of right ventricular dysfunction [6]. Intuitively, this observation is unsurprising, but it is poorly documented in terms of the influence of pulmonary regurgitation. To test this premise more directly, my colleagues and I performed a series of studies in children and young adults at the time of cardiac catheterization [7]. Using a conductance catheter, pulmonary regurgitation was measured beat-by-beat during balloon dilation and stenting of peripheral pulmonary artery stenosis. Following successful relief of stenosis, subsequent balloon inflation in the branch pulmonary artery was associated with a linear increase in the amount of pulmonary regurgitation. Although this simulated branch pulmonary artery stenosis led to the most profound changes in pulmonary regurgitation, the study also showed that the subtle waxing and waning in mean airway pressure associated with positive pressure ventilation also led to significant changes in pulmonary incompetence, independent of any pulmonary artery stenosis. Subtle pressure transients in the pulmonary vascular bed may lead to significant changes in the volume of pulmonary incompetence.

This phenomenon is further illustrated by a recent study from the Toronto group [8]. The total volume of regurgitation across the outflow tract was measured using cardiac MR in a series of patients late after repair. The individual branch pulmonary artery contribution to this total regurgitant flow was also assessed (Fig. 2). Interestingly, regurgitation from the left pulmonary artery predominated. Indeed, in some individuals, over 90% of the total regurgitant volume at the outflow tract was contributed by regurgitation from the left pulmonary artery. There are many potential explanations for this phenomenon. Purely anatomic reasons could not be invoked, because there was no relationship between size of the pulmonary artery and its regurgitant

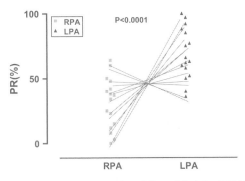

Fig. 2. Graph demonstrating differential right (RPA) and left pulmonary arterial (LPA) regurgitation as a percentage of the total regurgitant volume at the outflow tract. In some patients, over 80% of the total regurgitant volume is derived from the left pulmonary artery. (*Adapted from* Kang IS, Redington AN, Benson LN, et al. Differential regurgitation in branch pulmonary arteries after repair of tetralogy of Fallot: a phase-contrast cine magnetic resonance study. Circulation 2003;107(23):2940; with permission.)

volume. Although speculative, more subtle changes in the pulmonary vascular bed of the left lung may be responsible for the greater volume of regurgitation. It is easy to imagine a situation whereby some pulmonary incompetence leads to dilatation of the right ventricle, which increases the heart size, compressing the left lung. This increases its vascular impedance, generating more pulmonary incompetence and setting up a vicious spiral. The heart can be considered to be a "space-occupying lesion" under these circumstances.

*Ventricular diastolic performance*

Regurgitation into the ventricle will also be affected by its relaxation properties in early diastole, its compliance in late diastole, and, ultimately, its absolute capacitance. All of these properties may be abnormal in patients after repair of tetralogy of Fallot, and, clearly, all are subject to change with varying hemodynamic loads. There is a wide variability in right ventricular size (a reasonable surrogate of the total right ventricular volume load), even in the presence of a wide open outflow tract. Perhaps surprisingly, some patients, despite a transannular patch, fail to demonstrate significant right ventricular dilatation, suggesting the total hemodynamic burden as a result of free pulmonary incompetence is limited. Conversely, the majority of patients with identical outflow tract and pulmonary artery morphology will experience progressive right heart dilation under these circumstances.

The reason for these widely disparate responses must lie in the right ventricular diastolic performance. Indeed, my colleagues and I showed some years ago that the presence of restrictive right ventricular physiology limited the adverse effects of pulmonary incompetence [9]. The presence of antegrade diastolic flow, demonstrable by pulsed wave Doppler echocardiography in the distal pulmonary artery and pulmonary artery branches (Fig. 3), throughout respiration predicted a smaller right ventricular size, improved exercise performance, and lowered the propensity to arrhythmia [10]. Interestingly, this physiology when present in the early postoperative period was associated with worse outcome [11]. In the latter group, restrictive physiology was characterized by a lower cardiac output, a greater propensity to fluid retention, and a slower postoperative recovery. It remains unclear whether early postoperative restrictive physiology is the cause of late postoperative restrictive physiology, but an

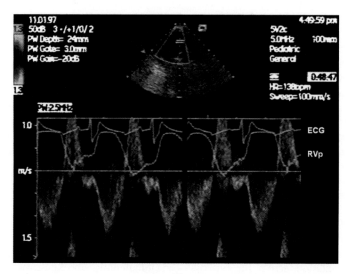

Fig. 3. Pulsed wave Doppler recording in the distal main pulmonary artery in a patient with restrictive right ventricular physiology. Note the antegrade late diastolic flow coincident with the p wave on the electrocardiogram (ECG). A micromanometer-tipped right ventricular pressure (RVp) recording is also displayed. Note the raised right ventricular end-diastolic pressure.

interesting study by Norgard and coworkers [12] showed that restrictive physiology in the early postoperative period was the only independent predictor of restriction at midterm follow-up.

The Doppler echocardiographic manifestations of restrictive right ventricular physiology are entirely qualitative. In essence, the presence of antegrade diastolic flow in the pulmonary artery reflects any situation in which the hydraulic impedance to blood flow into the pulmonary artery is lower than the resistance to filling of the right ventricle at end diastole. It is exquisitely variable with small changes in hemodynamics, not least the changes throughout the respiratory cycle. It may also be true that antegrade diastolic flow in the pulmonary artery appears when the right ventricle has dilated so much that its ultimate capacitance has been reached. Although highly significant as a group, not all patients with restrictive physiology have a small right ventricle. Indeed, there was considerable overlap in terms of right ventricular size and cardiothoracic ratio with the nonrestrictive group in our original series [10]. This finding might also explain some of the differences observed when "restrictive physiology" is diagnosed by Doppler echocardiography compared with cardiac MR imaging. Although several Doppler studies have confirmed our findings [13,14], some MR studies have suggested that the presence of restrictive physiology does not predict right ventricular size, function, or outcome. Furthermore, it has

recently been suggested that antegrade diastolic flow measured by magnetic resonance is associated with a worse outcome [15]. Although the reason for this disparity is not entirely clear, it should be remembered that MR measures antegrade diastolic flow as it is averaged throughout many respiratory and cardiac cycles. Furthermore, most measurements are made at the putative ventriculoarterial junction rather than the distal pulmonary artery. The orientation of the patient (lying flat on his or her back) may influence the pattern of flow in the proximal right ventricular outflow tract. All of these factors may conspire to make the interpretation of antegrade diastolic flow different when measured under these circumstances.

Regardless of the implications of antegrade diastolic flow, whether measured by Doppler echocardiography or MR imaging, the ultimate arbiter of outcome seems to be the amount of pulmonary incompetence and its effects on right ventricular size and performance. The measurement of pulmonary incompetence is crucial to the understanding of outcomes in these patients.

### Techniques for the measurement of pulmonary incompetence

#### Clinical surrogates

Although the presence of overt right heart dilatation clinically, a loud diastolic murmur, and signs of congestive cardiac failure represent one end of the hemodynamic spectrum, the assessment of pulmonary incompetence by clinical evaluation and auscultation cannot provide the detailed evaluation required for the longitudinal evaluation of these patients. Some useful simple outpatient investigations may provide a guide to severity. The utility of a chest radiograph should not be underestimated. In the absence of other hemodynamic contributors, a change of heart size on the chest radiograph may be a useful indicator of the presence of continued ventricular and atrial dilatation. In our original description of restrictive right ventricular physiology, patients with the smallest right ventricles by echocardiography had the smallest cardiothoracic ratios by chest radiography [9]. The cardiothoracic ratio is also a good generic predictor of overall functional performance. In an outstanding study of exercise performance in tetralogy of Fallot performed by the Chicago group [16], the cardiothoracic ratio was an important independent predictor of exercise performance. The smaller the heart size on the radiograph, the better the exercise performance in children and adolescents after surgery.

The electrocardiogram is also a reasonable surrogate measure of changes in right ventricular size. Reflecting the "mechano-electric" relationship, my colleagues and I showed some years ago that the QRS duration on the electrocardiogram is loosely related to right ventricular size measured by echocardiography [10]. Subsequently, this relationship has been confirmed in more elegant studies using MR assessment of right ventricular volume [17]. There can be no absolute guidelines regarding the relationship between QRS duration and right ventricular size because each patient has his or her own baseline QRS morphology and trajectories of change. Nonetheless, a significant change in the QRS duration is likely to reflect an important change in right ventricular size. Furthermore, a rapidly progressive prolongation of QRS duration is a harbinger of adverse clinical outcome in the form of ventricular arrhythmia and sudden death [18].

Although these surrogate measures may have some use in the outpatient assessment of patients, they clearly cannot be used for more sophisticated analysis of outcomes. For this alternative, more sensitive methods are required.

*Cardiac catheterization: conductance assessment of right ventricular volumes*

The subjective assessment of pulmonary incompetence from pulmonary arteriography and right ventriculography is clearly a thing of the past. Nonetheless, initial measurements of right ventricular pressure-volume relationships using digitized ventriculograms provide an improved understanding of the relationship between pulmonary incompetence and right ventricular hemodynamics [19]. Subsequently, the author and others have used conductance catheterization to assess right ventricular hemodynamics on a beat-by-beat basis [20,21]. This technique relies on the time varying change in blood pool resistance that is proportional to right ventricular volume as it changes throughout the cardiac cycle. A specialized catheter incorporating multiple electrodes is used to set up a series of electric fields within the ventricle. If the resistivity of blood is known, right ventricular size can be calculated from the composite change in blood conductance. This technique has a remarkably high temporal resolution (200 Hz) and can be combined with micromanometric pressure recordings to construct ventricular pressure-volume relationships from which the volume of pulmonary incompetence occurring during isovolumic relaxation can be measured. In patients with pulmonary regurgitation, right ventricular volume begins to increase well before the point of tricuspid valve opening. Assuming there is no residual ventricular septal defect or other source of volume increase in the ventricle during that period, the source must be via the pulmonary valve. The increase in volume between minimum (end systolic) volume and that at the time of tricuspid valve opening can be expressed as an index of pulmonary regurgitant volume [7,18]. The regurgitant volume measured in this way has been shown to relate to right ventricular end diastolic and end systolic size [7], to reflect differences in exercise performance [19], and, as mentioned previously, has been used to show the instantaneous change in pulmonary incompetence as right ventricular afterload increases [18]. It remains a useful experimental technique for the analysis of pulmonary incompetence in patients and in experimental models if instantaneous changes need to be measured. It would be foolish to suggest that this technique could be used clinically, because there are clearly far more satisfactory methods for general screening and longitudinal assessment.

*Cross-sectional echocardiography: Doppler assessment*

In general, the assessment of pulmonary incompetence by ultrasound techniques has been qualitative rather than quantitative. A variety of methods have been proposed [22], including the measurement of jet widths, the propagation of regurgitant color flow maps, and determination of the extent of regurgitation into the distal pulmonary arteries. Although all of these methods show some relationship to the true regurgitant volume, none can be used to assess small changes longitudinally. Indeed, it is likely that the experienced echocardiographer incorporates all of these patterns into a qualitative assessment of the severity of pulmonary incompetence. The size of the right ventricle, the appearance of the outflow tract and pulmonary arteries, and the Doppler patterns all are incorporated into the grading of severity.

Recently, an attempt at quantitation with comparison using MR imaging as a gold standard has been proposed. The pulmonary regurgitation index is a measure of pulmonary regurgitation severity based on the duration of the regurgitant signal by spectral Doppler study compared with the diastolic filling time. When this ratio is less than 0.77, Li and coworkers [23] suggest 100% sensitivity and 84% specificity for identifying patients with a pulmonary regurgitant fraction of greater than approximately 25% by MR imaging. Fig. 4 shows two patients with a similar pulmonary regurgitation index; both indices are significantly lower than the 0.77 cut-off suggested by Li and coworkers. Patient 1 had a normal right

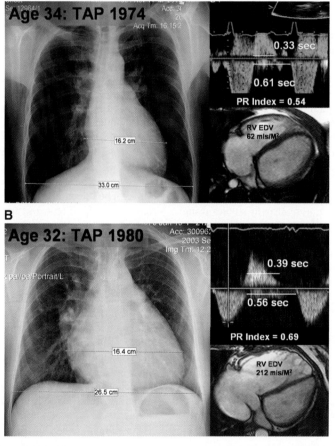

Fig. 4. Composite illustrations taken from two patients with a similar pulmonary regurgitation (PR) index (see text for details). In both cases, the index is predictive of severe PR; however, patient 1 (*A*) has a normal right ventricular size and little PR by MR imaging despite "free" pulmonary incompetence as a result of a transannular patch placed 20 years previously. This patient has restrictive right ventricular physiology that limits PR and prevents secondary dilation. Patient 2 (*B*) does have severe right ventricular volume overload and severe PR (and, paradoxically, a less severe PR index). These cases emphasize the need to be cautious with Doppler-derived surrogates of pulmonary incompetence in the individual patient.

ventricular size and only a small pulmonary regurgitant volume. This patient had a severely restrictive right ventricle. Patient 2 complied with the hypothesis that a low pulmonary regurgitation index is associated with severe pulmonary incompetence. MR imaging confirmed a huge right ventricle with a large pulmonary regurgitant volume. These findings suggest that the pulmonary regurgitant index should be used with caution.

There are two important pitfalls regarding use of the index. First, the presence of restrictive physiology, particularly if there is a variable or prolonged pulmonary regurgitant interval, will clearly influence this measurement in a counterintuitive way. Second, there is an increasing tendency to express pulmonary incompetence as a fraction or ratio of the total stroke volume. Indeed, the pulmonary regurgitant fraction is used in most of the MR-based studies of pulmonary incompetence nowadays. The use of the pulmonary regurgitant fraction is fundamentally flawed. Despite the relationship between the pulmonary regurgitant fraction and the absolute pulmonary regurgitant volume (which, in turn, will influence right ventricular size, hemodynamics, and so on), this relationship is variable. Patients who have relatively normal right ventricles and a relatively modest absolute volume of pulmonary regurgitant may have an identical regurgitant fraction to patients with a huge regurgitant volume and a proportionately larger right ventricular stroke volume.

My colleagues and I have recently looked at the relationship between the pulmonary regurgitant fraction and absolute pulmonary regurgitant volumes. In the graph shown in Fig. 5, it can be seen that, for the same pulmonary regurgitant fraction, the absolute volume of regurgitation may vary two or three fold. Conversely, for the same regurgitant volume, the pulmonary regurgitant fraction may vary markedly. Given that the measurement of absolute volume is one of the strengths of cardiac MR, it is disappointing that its application to the measurement of pulmonary incompetence has been simplified in this way. It is likely that absolute volume, when corrected for body surface area, for example, will prove to be a more robust parameter than the regurgitant fraction in the future.

*Cardiac magnetic resonance*

With the caveats expressed previously, cardiac MR is clearly the technique of choice when assessing pulmonary incompetence and right ventricular hemodynamics. Nonetheless, there are significant limitations to its use, and the lack of consistent protocols makes assessment of data from different groups difficult. Differences in sequencing and the types of signal generation affect the measurement of right ventricular volume and must be taken into account, even when following an individual patient longitudinally, as local equipment and protocols change.

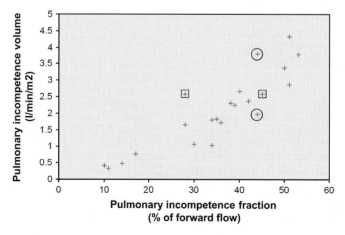

Fig. 5. Plot showing MR imaging–derived pulmonary regurgitant volume (corrected for body surface area) versus the pulmonary regurgitant fraction in individual patients. The patients highlighted in boxes have a similar regurgitant volume (2.5 L/min/m$^2$) but a regurgitant fraction of 28% and 47%, respectively. The circled patients have a similar regurgitant fraction of 42%, but one has double the pulmonary incompetence volume than the other (4 versus 2 L/min/m$^2$). The pulmonary regurgitant fraction does not adequately describe the preload on the right ventricle. (Unpublished data obtained in collaboration with Drs. Shi Joon Yoo and Lars Grosse-Wortmann, 2006.)

Furthermore, there remains a subjective element to right ventricular boundary recognition in terms of assessing the blood pool to myocardial interface and the right ventricular outflow tract. The latter is of particular significance. Frequently, these patients have grossly dilated, aneurysmal, and even dyskinetic segments of the outflow tract [24]. The junction between the ventricle and pulmonary artery is poorly defined and may vary from study to study and observer to observer. Frequently, the myocardial activity in the inlet and apical portions of the ventricle is far more vigorous than in the outflow tract. Whether independent measurements of function in the different areas may be of more utility, for example, in predicting reverse remodeling, remains to be seen. Despite the ability to measure directly pulmonary regurgitant volume for over a decade, we remain uncertain as to the clinical implications and utility of such measurements in terms of clinical decision making.

## Summary

Pulmonary incompetence is the single most important factor in the midterm outcome of patients after repair of tetralogy of Fallot. The pulmonary regurgitant volume and, hence, the burden on the right ventricle, is dependent on a subtle balance of orifice size, pulmonary afterload, and right ventricular diastolic physiology. Although the ability to measure pulmonary incompetence has improved significantly, there remain important pitfalls to its assessment in the individual patient, and our interpretation of its implications, regardless of which method is used, remains unsophisticated.

## References

[1] Anderson RH, Freedom RM. Normal and abnormal structure of the ventriculo-arterial junctions. Cardiol Young 2005;15(Suppl 1):3–16.

[2] Kirklin JW, Blackstone EH, Pacifico AD, et al. Risk factors for early and late failure after repair of tetralogy of Fallot, and their neutralization. Thorac Cardiovasc Surg 1984;32(4):208–14.

[3] Antunes MJ, Castela E, Sanches MF, et al. Preservation of the pulmonary annulus in total correction of tetralogy of Fallot: decreasing transannular gradients in the early follow-up period. Eur J Cardiothorac Surg 1991;5(10):528–32.

[4] Van Arsdell G, Yun TJ. An apology for primary repair of tetralogy of Fallot. Semin Thorac Cardiovasc Surg Pediatr Card Surg Annu 2005;128–31.

[5] Pigula FA, Khalil PN, Mayer JE, et al. Repair of tetralogy of Fallot in neonates and young infants. Circulation 1999;100(19 Suppl):II157–61.

[6] Sunakawa A, Shirotani H, Yokoyama T, et al. Factors affecting biventricular function following surgical repair of tetralogy of Fallot. Jpn Circ J 1988;52(5):401–10.

[7] Chaturvedi RR, Kilner PJ, White PA, et al. Increased airway pressure and simulated branch pulmonary artery stenosis increase pulmonary regurgitation after repair of tetralogy of Fallot: real-time analysis with a conductance catheter technique. Circulation 1997;95(3):643–9.

[8] Kang IS, Redington AN, Benson LN, et al. Differential regurgitation in branch pulmonary arteries after repair of tetralogy of Fallot: a phase-contrast cine magnetic resonance study. Circulation 2003;107(23):2938–43.

[9] Gatzoulis MA, Clark AL, Cullen S, et al. Right ventricular diastolic function 15 to 35 years after repair of tetralogy of Fallot: restrictive physiology predicts superior exercise performance. Circulation 1995; 91(6):1775–81.

[10] Gatzoulis MA, Till JA, Somerville J, et al. Mechanoelectrical interaction in tetralogy of Fallot: QRS prolongation relates to right ventricular size and predicts malignant ventricular arrhythmias and sudden death. Circulation 1995;92(2):231–7.

[11] Cullen S, Shore D, Redington A. Characterization of right ventricular diastolic performance after complete repair of tetralogy of Fallot: restrictive physiology predicts slow postoperative recovery. Circulation 1995;91(6):1782–9.

[12] Norgard G, Gatzoulis MA, Josen M, et al. Does restrictive right ventricular physiology in the early postoperative period predict subsequent right ventricular restriction after repair of tetralogy of Fallot? Heart 1998;79(5):481–4.

[13] Sachdev MS, Bhagyavathy A, Varghese R, et al. Right ventricular diastolic function after repair of tetralogy of Fallot. Pediatr Cardiol 2006;27(2): 250–5.

[14] Eroglu AG, Sarioglu A, Sarioglu T. Right ventricular diastolic function after repair of tetralogy of Fallot: its relationship to the insertion of a "transannular" patch. Cardiol Young 1999;9(4):384–91.

[15] Helbing WA, Niezen RA, Le Cessie S, et al. Right ventricular diastolic function in children with pulmonary regurgitation after repair of tetralogy of Fallot: volumetric evaluation by magnetic resonance velocity mapping. J Am Coll Cardiol 1996;28(7): 1827–35.

[16] Wessel HU, Cunningham WJ, Paul MH, et al. Exercise performance in tetralogy of Fallot after intracardiac repair. J Thorac Cardiovasc Surg 1980;80(4): 582–93.

[17] Abd El Rahman MY, Abdul-Khaliq H, Vogel M, et al. Relation between right ventricular enlargement, QRS duration, and right ventricular function in patients with tetralogy of Fallot and pulmonary

regurgitation after surgical repair. Heart 2000;84(4):416–20.

[18] Gatzoulis MA, Balaji S, Webber SA, et al. Risk factors for arrhythmia and sudden cardiac death late after repair of tetralogy of Fallot: a multicentre study. Lancet 2000;356(9234):975–81.

[19] Redington AN, Oldershaw PJ, Shinebourne EA, et al. A new technique for the assessment of pulmonary regurgitation and its application to the assessment of right ventricular function before and after repair of tetralogy of Fallot. Br Heart J 1988;60(1):57–65.

[20] Dickstein ML, Yano O, Spotnitz HM, et al. Assessment of right ventricular contractile state with the conductance catheter technique in the pig. Cardiovasc Res 1995;29(6):820–6.

[21] Lambermont B, Ghuysen A, Kolh P, et al. Effects of endotoxic shock on right ventricular systolic function and mechanical efficiency. Cardiovasc Res 2003;59(2):412–8.

[22] Mulhern KM, Skorton DJ. Echocardiographic evaluation of isolated pulmonary valve disease in adolescents and adults. Echocardiography 1993;10(5):533–43.

[23] Li W, Davlouros PA, Kilner PJ, et al. Doppler-echocardiographic assessment of pulmonary regurgitation in adults with repaired tetralogy of Fallot: comparison with cardiovascular magnetic resonance imaging. Am Heart J 2004;147(1):165–72.

[24] Davlouros PA, Kilner PJ, Hornung TS, et al. Right ventricular function in adults with repaired tetralogy of Fallot assessed with cardiovascular magnetic resonance imaging: detrimental role of right ventricular outflow aneurysms or akinesia and adverse right-to-left ventricular interaction. J Am Coll Cardiol 2002;40(11):2044–52.

ELSEVIER
SAUNDERS

CARDIOLOGY
CLINICS

Cardiol Clin 24 (2006) 641–660

# Exercise Intolerance in Adults with Congenital Heart Disease

Konstantinos Dimopoulos, MD[a,b,*], Gerhard-Paul Diller, MD[a,b],
Massimo F. Piepoli, MD, PhD[b], Michael A. Gatzoulis, MD, PhD, FACC[a]

[a]Adult Congenital Heart Programme, Department of Cardiology, Royal Brompton Hospital,
Sydney Street, London, UK
[b]Department of Clinical Cardiology, National Heart and Lung Institute, Imperial College School of Medicine,
London, SW3 6NP, UK

Exercise intolerance is a common feature of congenital and acquired heart disease. It affects approximately one third of adults with congenital heart disease (CHD) and is present in all congenital groups, including those with simple lesions [1]. Its clinical manifestations are exertional dyspnea or exertional fatigue, and it is one of the most frequent causes of reduced quality of life in adult CHD (ACHD) [2–4].

CHD shares important features with heart failure in patients with acquired heart disease, both in the clinical presentation and systemic manifestations. CHD is, in fact, a cause of the so-called heart failure syndrome. Traditionally, heart failure was identified with left ventricular systolic dysfunction of idiopathic or ischemic origin. Recent American College of Cardiology/American Heart Association (ACC/AHA) and European Society of Cardiology guidelines define heart failure mainly on the basis of symptoms of exercise intolerance and recognize it can be caused by various cardiac disorders beyond left ventricular systolic dysfunction [5,6]. It has become apparent that heart failure is a clinical syndrome with numerous systemic manifestations and multiple potential causes, including CHD.

This article describes the ways to assess exercise capacity in CHD and the impact of exercise intolerance in the ACHD population. It also discusses the likely pathogenesis of exercise intolerance in CHD, the similarities between ACHD and acquired heart failure, and potential therapeutic options.

## Assessment of exercise intolerance in the adult congenital heart disease population

### Subjective assessment

The most popular means of quantification of physical impairment in ACHD is the New York Heart Association (NYHA) classification [3,4]. It is an established semiquantitative means of subjective assessment of the degree of exercise intolerance in chronic heart failure. The NYHA classification has been adopted by ACHD health providers, because it is easy to use and is familiar to health workers outside the area of ACHD [7]. It is also often reported (inappropriately) as a measure of health-related quality of life in ACHD despite the existence of other specific scoring systems of ACHD quality of life [3,4,8].

### Objective assessment

#### Cardiopulmonary exercise testing

Cardiopulmonary exercise testing is a powerful tool for the simultaneous objective evaluation of

K.D. has been supported by the European Society of Cardiology. G-P.D. is supported by Actelion, UK. The Royal Brompton Adult Congenital Heart Program and the Department of Clinical Cardiology have received support from the British Heart Foundation and the Clinical Research Committee, Royal Brompton Hospital, London.

* Corresponding author.

*E-mail address:* k.dimopoulos@ic.ac.uk
(K. Dimopoulos).

the cardiovascular, respiratory, and muscular systems under conditions of controlled metabolic stress [9]. It is used widely for assessing patients with acquired heart failure, and, like the NYHA classification, it has been adopted by ACHD physicians, gradually becoming part of the routine clinical assessment of ACHD patients. Incremental protocols are used to assess important prognostic indices such as peak oxygen consumption (peak VO$_2$), ventilatory response to exercise, anaerobic threshold, and heart rate response [10].

Peak VO$_2$ is the highest measured value of oxygen uptake (usually expressed in mL/kg/min) and approximates the maximal aerobic power of each individual (Fig. 1) [11,12]. It is a surrogate of the functional status of the pulmonary, cardio–circulatory, and muscular systems and represents the upper limit of oxygen use. It is the most frequently reported exercise parameter because of its simplicity and prognostic power both in acquired heart disease and in ACHD. Peak VO$_2$ approximates maximal exercise capacity to the extent that the patient is able and determined to exercise to exhaustion. When patients fail to exercise to the maximum of their capacity, measured peak VO$_2$ will not reflect their true exercise capacity. Moreover, as it is derived only

from few measurements at peak exercise, it can be prone to technical error [13].

The anaerobic threshold is the level of oxygen consumption above which aerobic metabolism is supplemented by anaerobic processes [10,11,13]. Above the anaerobic threshold, lactate accumulates and is buffered by plasma bicarbonate, causing an increase in carbon dioxide (CO$_2$) production (VCO$_2$). Recognition of the anaerobic threshold is achieved by observing the VCO$_2$ versus VO$_2$ slope (the V-slope method) or the ventilation versus VO$_2$ and VCO$_2$ slopes (the ventilatory equivalent method) [11]. The anaerobic threshold carries important pathophysiologic and prognostic information in acquired heart failure [14]. Nevertheless, in more symptomatic patients, its recognition can be difficult, despite the development of automated algorithms [13].

The VE/VCO$_2$ slope is the slope of the regression line between minute ventilation (VE) and VCO$_2$ (Fig. 2) and has been proposed as an exercise parameter that is independent of achieving maximal exertion. It is a simplification of the complex relation between ventilation and VCO$_2$ and appears to contain important physiological and prognostic information [14,15]. It is easy to calculate, is highly reproducible, and is a marker

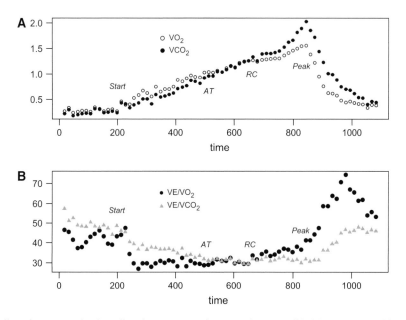

Fig. 1. Recordings from a maximal cardiopulmonary exercise test using a modified Bruce protocol in a patient after Fontan-type operation. (*A*) Oxygen consumption (VO$_2$) and carbon dioxide production (VCO$_2$ in mL/min) as related to time (in seconds). (*B*) The ratio VE/VO$_2$ and VE/VCO$_2$ against time. Abbreviations: AT, anaerobic threshold; Peak, peak exercise; RC, respiratory compensation point; Start, start exercise; VE, ventilation.

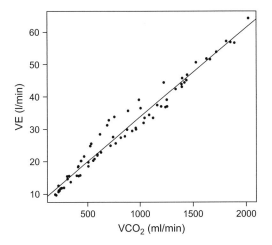

Fig. 2. Plot of ventilation (VE) versus $VCO_2$ from the same patient as Fig. 1. The $VE/VCO_2$ slope is the slope of the regression line between ventilation (VE) and $VCO_2$ (*continuous line*). This can be calculated either over the entire duration of exercise (as shown in this figure), or after exclusion of the portion following the respiratory compensation point [16]. In this case, using data from the entire period of exercise, the $VE/VCO_2$ slope is 28, suggesting that no ventilatory inefficiency is present.

of exercise intolerance strongly related to peak $VO_2$ and to mortality in acquired heart failure [14,15]. The mechanism behind the abnormal ventilatory response to increments in $CO_2$ production is not yet understood fully. Several mechanisms have been proposed, such as pulmonary hypoperfusion or vasoconstriction with increased physiological dead space and ventilation/perfusion mismatch and stimulation of the respiratory centers by triggers other than $CO_2$ [16]. It is generally recommended that the nonlinear portion of the VE versus $VCO_2$ relation at the start of exercise and after the respiratory compensation point (the point at which hyperventilation occurs in response to increasing lactate production) should be excluded when calculating the $VE/VCO_2$ slope. Nevertheless, numerous studies that have established $VE/VCO_2$ as an important exercise parameter have not used this theoretically appealing convention [15,17,18]. One study on patients with acquired heart failure has suggested that the $VE/VCO_2$ slope calculated using the entire exercise period is prognostically stronger [19]. In the authors' center, the $VE/VCO_2$ slope is routinely calculated as an adjunct to peak $VO_2$ in assessing exercise capacity and prognosis in the ACHD population (Fig. 3). Values of $VE/VCO_2$ slope

exceeding 33 are considered abnormal. In noncyanotic patients who have ACHD, a $VE/VCO_2$ slope of 38 or above identifies those at a 10-fold increased risk of mortality at a mean follow-up of 20 months (Fig. 4) [16].

*6-minute-walk test*

The 6-minute walk test is a submaximal timed distance test often employed in patients who have ACHD. The main response variable in this type of exercise testing is the distance that individuals are able to cover at their own pace in 6 minutes. A normal 40-year-old subject covers approximately 600 m, decreasing by 50 m per decade [20]. Oxygen saturations by portable pulse oximetry can also be recorded.

The 6-min walk test reflects ordinary daily activities and is easy to perform. It is a submaximal test in healthy individuals and mildly impaired patients but can be a maximal test in highly symptomatic patients. Indeed, the 6-minute walking test distance correlated well to peak $VO_2$ in a study of highly symptomatic patients [21]. It is commonly used to assess the response to advanced therapies in patients with pulmonary hypertension and is the only test approved by the US Food and Drug Administration (FDA) as an endpoint for prospective clinical trials in this population [22,23]. Correlation to peak $VO_2$ appears to be best when distance is adjusted for patient weight (distance × weight) [24].

It may be inappropriate to use the 6-min walk test in patients with mild impairment of exercise capacity, because it could mask improvement after an intervention [25]. Reproducibility and comparability of repeated 6-min walking tests also depend on adequate standardization of the protocol used. An important learning effect has also been described and should be considered when comparing the first with subsequent tests [26].

## Exercise intolerance in adult patients with congenital heart disease

The Euro Heart Survey, a large European registry of ACHD patients reported that approximately one third of ACHD patients complain of symptoms of exercise intolerance (Fig. 5) [1]. Patients with cyanotic lesions and those with univentricular hearts have the highest prevalence of exercise intolerance, whereas patients with aortic coarctation are usually asymptomatic [1,27,28]. Eisenmenger patients have by far the

**Royal Brompton & Harefield** **NHS**

NHS Trust

Non-invasive Cardiology Sydney Street, London, SW3 6NP

Cardiopulmonary Exercise Testing with Respiratory Gas Analysis (MVO2)

## Surname, Name

RBH 5567
14-Nov-1972
M
Ebstein's anomaly of the TV
III NYHA
168 cm
52 kg

| | |
|---|---|
| conducted on | 23-Dec-2005 |
| Exercise duration | 12 min 34 sec |

RER — 1.12

PeakVO$_2$ — **17.3** ml/kg/min

*Predicted MVO2* — 31 ml/kg/min

VE/VCO$_2$ slope — **61.0**

Anaerobic Threshold — **11.0** ml/kg/min

| | | | | |
|---|---|---|---|---|
| Rhythm | SR | | | |
| Resting pulse | 73 | BP | 105 | / 70 |
| Peak Exercise pulse | 148 | BP | 170 | / 85 |
| Limiting symptom | Dyspnoea | | | |

COMMENTS

Peak VO2 of 17.3ml/kg/min is 56% of predicted. Significantly increased VE/VCO2 slope of 61 indicates reduced ventilatory efficiency. Appropriate blood pressure response, suboptimal chronotropic response to exercise. Resting O2 sats of 96%, decreased to 85% at peak exercise.

SPIROMETRY

| | | | | |
|---|---|---|---|---|
| FEV1 | 2.7 l | 78.0% of pred | Operator | Supervising physician |
| FVC | 2.9 l | 70.0% of pred | | |
| PEF | 357 l/min | | | Room C |

Fig. 3. Example of the form used at the authors' center for reporting cardiopulmonary exercise tests. Peak VO$_2$, the VE/VCO$_2$ slope, blood pressure and heart rate response, and oxygen saturation at rest and during exercise are reported routinely.

highest degree of subjective impairment, suggesting a synergistic detrimental effect of cyanosis and pulmonary hypertension. In one cohort of 188 patients with this condition, 68% were symptomatic by age 9, rising to 84% at age 28 [29]. Marked exercise intolerance also has been reported in patients who have congenitally corrected (l-) transposition of the great arteries [30,31]. Similarly, patients after atrial switch for transposition of the great arteries are symptomatic with exertional dyspnea, whereas those with repaired tetralogy of Fallot are generally less limited in their exercise capacity [32–34].

Significant objective impairment in exercise capacity has been described in various ACHD groups using cardiopulmonary exercise testing [18,35–43]. In the authors' laboratory, routine cardiopulmonary exercise testing applied to a large cohort of ACHD patients provided estimates of exercise capacity across the spectrum of CHD (Fig. 6) [44]. Peak VO$_2$ was depressed in all ACHD groups compared with healthy subjects of similar age, but varied according to underlying anatomy. Peak heart rate, forced expiratory volume (%FEV1), pulmonary arterial hypertension, cyanosis, gender, and body mass index were independent predictors of peak VO$_2$ in this population. Systemic and pulmonary ventricular function were not predictive of peak VO$_2$ on multivariate analysis, confirming in ACHD what is already known in acquired heart failure, that exercise capacity is independent of resting cardiac function [45,46].

The subjective assessment of exercise intolerance using the NYHA classification appears to underestimate the severity of functional

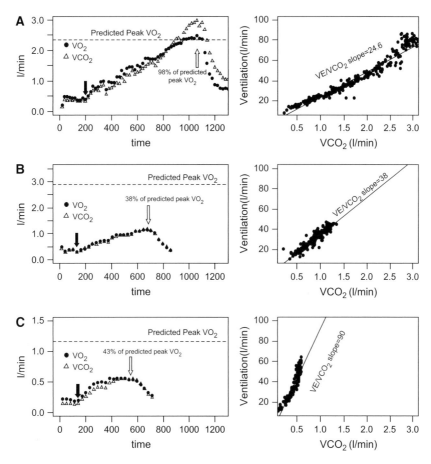

Fig. 4. Examples of cardiopulmonary exercise tests. (*A*) An asymptomatic (NYHA class I) 40-year-old patient with repaired tetralogy of Fallot underwent cardiopulmonary exercise testing as part of routine clinical assessment. Peak $VO_2$ was 29 mL/kg/min. This was calculated as the mean of the two highest consecutive values of 15-second averages of $VO_2$ divided by the patient's weight (in this case 2450 mL/min divided by 84 kg of weight) and was 98% of predicted for age, weight, height, and gender. The $VE/VCO_2$ slope was 24.6, within normal limits. He had an adequate heart rate (90 to 171 bpm) and blood pressure response (118/78 to 158/92 mm Hg). No desaturation was observed. In this case, cardiopulmonary exercise testing confirmed an optimal exercise tolerance. (*B*) Mildly symptomatic (NYHA class II) 20-year-old man after Fontan-type operation. He exercised for 8.6 min and reached a peak $VO_2$ of 16.8 mL/kg/min, which was 38% of predicted. The $VE/VCO_2$ slope was 38, which is abnormally raised. Blood pressure and heart rate response were blunted (80 to 133 bpm and 100/64 to 132/72mm Hg). No desaturation was observed, making right-to-left shunting (commonly observed in Fontan patients) unlikely. The results of the exercise test suggest that this patient had an exercise capacity that was impaired significantly, more than what was suggested by his symptoms. This patient was found to have moderate-to-severe systemic ventricular dysfunction. Moreover, a peak $VO_2$ of less than 15.5 mL/kg/min and $VE/VCO_2$ slope of 38 would identify this patient, in retrospect, at high risk of hospitalization and death, which was indeed the case [16,44]. The patient died 6 months after the index exercise test. (*C*) A mildly symptomatic 52-year-old woman with Eisenmenger physiology. She exercised for 6.3 minutes and reached a peak $VO_2$ of 11.2 mL/kg/min, which was 43% of predicted. The $VE/VCO_2$ slope was 90, which is severely raised. Her resting saturations were 90% and decreased to 45% at peak exercise, when she became light-headed and had to stop. Heart rate response was appropriate (89 to 151 bpm), but blood pressure response was suboptimal (128/82 to 142/80mm Hg). In this case, the cardiopulmonary exercise test revealed significant exercise intolerance and severe ventilatory inefficiency. Despite near-normal resting oxygen saturations, severe desaturation occurred and was likely the cause of termination of exercise. Moreover, the significant right-to-left shunt likely caused a significant ventilation-perfusion (V/Q) mismatch and stimulation of peripheral and central chemoreceptors, leading to an increase in ventilation, disproportionate to $CO_2$ production.

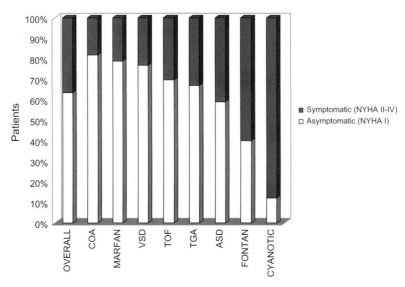

Fig. 5. Symptomatic (NYHA class II or more) versus asymptomatic (NYHA class I) ACHD patients according to underlying anatomy. (*Data from* Engelfiet P, Boersma E, Oechslin E, et al. The spectrum of adult congenital heart disease in Europe: morbidity and mortality in a 5-year follow-up period. The Euro Heart Survey on adult congenital heart disease. Eur Heart J 2005;26(21):2325–33.)

impairment in ACHD. A linear relationship exists between NYHA class and peak $VO_2$ across the spectrum of ACHD, but many asymptomatic ACHD patients show dramatically lower peak $VO_2$ values compared with normal controls. Use of a subjective measure like NYHA class, which is based on the perception of ordinary everyday activity in a population of patients with inborn heart defects, understandably leads to underestimation of the real degree of impairment. This appears to be an important point of disparity between ACHD and acquired heart failure, in which the difference in peak $VO_2$ between normal controls and asymptomatic heart failure patients is much less. Peak $VO_2$ values of ACHD patients in the authors' study approximated those of older patients with acquired heart failure and similar NYHA class. Subjective assessment using the NYHA classification thus seems to adequately categorize ACHD patients into classes of decreasing exercise capacity but cannot be used to assess the magnitude of exercise intolerance in this population. This underlines the importance of cardiopulmonary exercise testing for the routine clinical assessment of patients with ACHD [44,47].

The authors recently described abnormally high mean values of the $VE/VCO_2$ slope in all major ACHD groups compared with normal controls [16]. The Eisenmenger and complex diagnoses groups were found to have the highest $VE/VCO_2$ slopes. Cyanosis was the strongest independent predictor of the $VE/VCO_2$ slope in this cohort and appeared to have a significant impact on the ventilatory response to exercise. The $VE/VCO_2$ slope showed a linear relation to NYHA class, suggesting a link between the ventilatory response to exercise and the occurrence of symptoms. The $VE/VCO_2$ slope was raised significantly even among asymptomatic patients, further underscoring the importance of objective assessment of exercise capacity in ACHD.

## Mechanisms of reduced exercise capacity in adult congenital heart disease

*The components of exercise: the lungs, the heart, the blood, the vessels, and the skeletal muscles*

During exercise, skeletal muscles must regenerate energy continuously in the form of ATP [48]. Aerobic metabolism is by far the most efficient means of ATP production, but it requires adequate coupling of external respiration (oxygen delivery) to cellular respiration (muscle requirements). Anaerobic glycolysis becomes active when oxygen delivery is inadequate. It requires no oxygen but produces smaller amounts of ATP and has lactic acid as a by-product, which

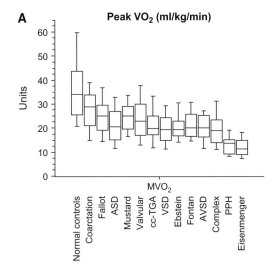

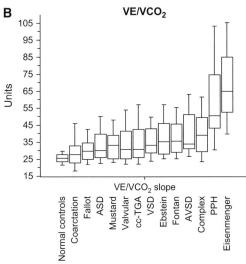

Fig. 6. Peak VO$_2$ and VE/VCO$_2$ slope in various ACHD groups. Data on 933 ACHD patients and controls from the Royal Brompton Hospital cardiopulmonary exercise testing laboratory. ASD, atrial septal defect; AVSD, atrioventricular septal defect; cc-TGA, congenitally corrected (l-) transposition of the great arteries; Complex, complex anatomy (double inlet or outlet right and left ventricle or complex pulmonary atresia); PPH, idiopathic pulmonary arterial hypertension; VSD, ventricular septal defect.

is buffered by bicarbonate, generating CO$_2$. The hydrolysis of phosphocreatine is another anaerobic mechanism of ATP production, which becomes transiently active at the beginning of exercise, when the circulation has not had time to respond to the activity of the muscles [9,48].

Exercise capacity largely depends on adequate coupling of muscle and external respiration (ie, on an adequate delivery of oxygen to meet the needs of the active muscles and sustain the aerobic regeneration of ATP). Adequate oxygen supply depends on a chain of events: ventilation, lung perfusion, and the cardiovascular system. Abnormalities in any of these elements (lungs, heart, blood, blood vessels) can be detrimental and limit exercise capacity. CHD can affect all components of the cardiorespiratory chain, resulting in a significant impairment of exercise capacity.

*The heart*

The heart plays a key role in metabolic–respiratory coupling during exercise. An adequate increase in systemic cardiac output is essential to meet the metabolic demands of the working muscles. The heart increases its output by increments in stroke volume and heart rate. The left ventricle is directly responsible for the increase in systemic cardiac output but can only achieve this in the presence of an adequate increment in right ventricular output. At the start of exercise, pulmonary vascular resistance drops, allowing the right ventricle to increase pulmonary perfusion and blood to return to the left ventricle. Moreover, significant ventricular interaction occurs in CHD, especially in cases of right ventricular overload such as Ebstein's anomaly [49]. Thus, conditions that affect the left or the right ventricle can have a great impact on exercise capacity [50].

Most types of CHD impart a hemodynamic load (pressure or volume overload) upon one or both ventricles. This load is, by definition in congenital heart disease, long-standing and can lead to severe ventricular dysfunction. Significant impairment of systemic ventricular function was found 10 to 30 years after surgery in patients after atrial repair of transposition of the great arteries, congenitally corrected transposition of the great arteries, and patients with Fontan-like circulations [27,30,31,51–57].

Right ventricular systolic dysfunction is typically present in Ebstein's anomaly and in patients who have arrhythmogenic right ventricular dysplasia [58,59]. Moreover, significant pulmonary regurgitation after repair of tetralogy of Fallot or of isolated pulmonary stenosis can also lead to right ventricular dysfunction, as can other causes of right ventricular volume or pressure overload (atrial septal defects, atrioventricular septal defects with tricuspid regurgitation, pulmonary stenosis, or Eisenmenger physiology) [50,58]. Finally, it has been observed that repeated operations involving protracted cardiopulmonary bypass, especially those performed in previous eras, and right ventricular outflow tract patch augmentation, can affect right ventricular function adversely [50,58,60].

*Arrhythmias*

Patients who have ACHD have an increased propensity to arrhythmias. This can be attributed to several factors such as the congenital cardiac lesion itself, long-standing hemodynamic factors, and scarring from previous surgery. Arrhythmias in ACHD will often cause cardiac dysfunction and may become life-threatening, especially when very fast, when of ventricular origin, or in the presence of significant underlying disease. Nevertheless, even supraventricular tachycardias with a mild increase in ventricular rate can cause a reduction in cardiac output because of loss of atrioventricular synchrony or when long-standing. Li and colleagues showed that patients who have ACHD with atrial flutter (mean ventricular rate 106 plus or minus 21bpm) developed a dramatically decreased exercise duration and lower peak blood pressure and systemic ventricular function [61]. The authors have reported that patients in sinus rhythm during cardiopulmonary exercise testing have a higher peak heart rate and a higher peak $VO_2$ compared with those not in sinus rhythm [44]. Tachycardia management in ACHD remains challenging because of complex and variable hemodynamic profiles, extensive scarring from prior surgery, and anatomical variance posing ongoing difficulties to electrical therapies.

*Chronotropic incompetence*

Cardiac output is the product of stroke volume and heart rate. Stroke volume increases at the beginning of exercise, whereas further increments in cardiac output occur through increases in heart rate. Chronotropic incompetence is the inability of the heart rate to increase appropriate to the metabolic demands during exercise and can be a cause of exercise intolerance [62]. Even though the concept of chronotropic incompetence appears straight-forward, a definition of normal or expected heart rate response to exercise is elusive. Numerous formulas have been proposed, the most widely used being 220 minus age or the Astrand formula [63].

In acquired heart failure, chronotropic incompetence relates to NYHA class and peak $VO_2$ [64]. Moreover, chronotropic incompetence is a predictor of adverse outcome in patients with ischemic heart disease and in the general population [65–67]. In the ACHD population, chronotropic incompetence is also prevalent and relates to exercise capacity [37,68,69]. The authors recently reported that heart rate reserve (HRR equals peak heart rate minus resting heart rate) is a strong predictor of mortality, especially in patients who have complex lesions, Fontan-type surgery, and repaired tetralogy of Fallot [70]. Whether the prognostic power of HRR is the result of its relationship to autonomic imbalance and exercise capacity needs to be elucidated [71,72].

*Pacing*

Pacemaker therapy has an important role for managing patients who have ACHD. Sinus node dysfunction is present in 13% to 44% of patients after Fontan operation and in 50% of patients after atrial switch repair for transposition of the great arteries [73]. Atrioventricular block used to be common immediately after surgical repair of perimembranous or infundibular ventricular septal defects or after right ventricular muscle bundle resection. It can also develop later in life, irrespective of surgery, in patients who have atrioventricular septal defects and congenitally corrected (l-) transposition [73]. Right ventricular pacing can cause ventricular asynchrony, and in the noncongenital population, it has been shown to cause left ventricular dysfunction and reduced exercise capacity [74–76]. Dual-chamber pacemakers are being implanted increasingly, maintaining atrioventricular synchrony in an attempt to optimize ventricular function and cardiac output [77]. Although rate-responsive pacemakers are used almost universally, rate responsiveness at higher levels of exercise may be inadequate to maintain an adequate cardiac output. In the authors' experience, ACHD patients with permanent pacemakers have significantly lower values of peak heart rate and a trend toward lower peak $VO_2$ compared with those without a pacemaker [44].

*Myocardial perfusion abnormalities*

Myocardial perfusion is a major determinant of ventricular function. Abnormal myocardial perfusion has been suggested as an underlying cause of ventricular dysfunction in CHD. Reversible and fixed perfusion defects with concordant regional wall motion abnormalities and impaired myocardial flow reserve often occur in the right ventricle of patients with transposition of the great arteries long after atrial repair [53,78]. Myocardial perfusion defects are also common in patients after an arterial switch operation [79–81]. These perfusion abnormalities correlate well to impaired ventricular function and are seen more frequently in older patients with longer follow-up. Although the genesis of these abnormalities remains obscure, it is likely that myocardial perfusion defects may be a sensitive predictor of systemic ventricular impairment and a target for future therapies [52,57,82–86].

*Pericardial disease*

Previous cardiac surgery for congenital or acquired disease is a known risk factor for developing constrictive pericarditis. This is a rare disease, occurring in approximately 0.2% of operated patients [87]. Constrictive pericarditis can have dramatic effects, causing significant exercise intolerance and signs of congestive heart failure. Diagnosis requires a high degree of suspicion and has to be part of the differential diagnosis of unexplained exercise intolerance, especially when dealing with the ACHD population in which most patients have undergone cardiac surgery [87,88].

Partial and total absence of the pericardium can also cause significant changes in cardiac anatomy and compromise cardiac function. Loss of the pericardial constraint can result in ventricular dilation in response to small increases in preload [89,90]. Disruption of the anatomy of the tricuspid valve can lead to severe tricuspid regurgitation and significant right ventricular dilation [91–93]. Pericardial absence can affect systemic venous return, and, to a minor extent, pulmonary venous return [94]. Finally, total absence of the pericardium is associated with abnormal interventricular septal movement, which relates to left ventricular rotation and motion abnormality [95].

*Medication*

Beta-blockers, calcium antagonists, and anti-arrhythmic drugs with negative inotropic and chronotropic effects are often used in ACHD and can affect ventricular performance and exercise capacity. In the authors' experience ACHD patients on beta-blocker therapy have a lower peak heart rate during maximal exercise testing and lower peak $VO_2$ than patients not on beta-blockers [44]. Underlying conduction system disease is often latent in patients who have ACHD, and medication can unmask sinus node dysfunction, atrioventricular block, and chronotropic incompetence [96]. Particular care and close follow-up are thus needed when such therapies are prescribed in this population.

### Other conditions that can affect exercise capacity

*Cyanosis, pulmonary vascular disease, and Eisenmenger physiology*

Cyanosis and pulmonary hypertension significantly affect exercise capacity. Objective data confirm that Eisenmenger and complex patients with cyanosis are impaired significantly in their ability to exercise [1,17]. The effect of right-to-left shunting is obvious from the onset of exercise, when $VO_2$ fails to increase because of the inability to sufficiently increase pulmonary blood flow [8,97]. In these patients, an increase in cardiac output is obtained through shunting, at the expense of further systemic desaturation. An abrupt, exaggerated increase in ventilation occurs almost at the onset of exercise, resulting in alveolar hyperventilation, a rise in $VCO_2$ and a drop in $VO_2$ [97]. This accounts for the transient increase in the respiratory quotient (the ratio between $VCO_2$ and $VO_2$) often encountered in these patients at the start of exercise.

Although ventilation is increased, ventilatory efficiency is impaired significantly, as suggested by very high values of the $VE/VCO_2$ slope in cyanotic patients [16]. Pulmonary hypoperfusion, an increase in physiological dead-space through right-to-left shunting, and enhanced ventilatory reflex sensitivity are potential mechanisms contributing to the ventilatory inefficiency and the failure to meet oxygen requirements [16]. Although the inefficiency of the ventilatory response to exercise in cyanotic patients suggested by the $VE/VCO_2$ slope could lead to the early onset of dyspnea and exercise limitation, the exaggerated ventilatory response in these patients appears appropriate from a chemical point of view. In fact, hyperventilation succeeds in maintaining near-normal arterial $PCO_2$ and pH levels in the systemic circulation, at least during mild-to-moderate exertion, despite significant right-to-left shunting [40].

The effect of cyanosis on exercise capacity and ventilation is difficult to distinguish from that of pulmonary hypertension. Significant ventilatory inefficiency and a hyperventilatory response to exercise have been described in patients with primary pulmonary hypertension in the absence of right-to-left shunting [98,99]. The authors recently reported that patients with significant pulmonary hypertension and cyanosis have significantly higher $VE/VCO_2$ slopes compared with those without cyanosis, suggesting an additive effect of cyanosis on ventilation over that of pulmonary hypertension alone. Moreover, Fontan patients with cyanosis have higher $VE/VCO_2$ slopes compared with those without, suggesting a significant effect of cyanosis on ventilation even in the absence of pulmonary arterial hypertension [16].

*Anemia and secondary erythrocytosis*

Adequate blood oxygen carrying capacity is fundamental for the normal response to exercise. Hemoglobin carries oxygen and regulates the amount released at the tissue level [8,86]. Anemia results in reduced oxygen carrying capacity and a premature shift to anaerobic metabolism during exercise. In acquired chronic heart failure, anemia relates to exercise capacity and is a predictor of outcome. It is also known to precipitate heart failure, by affecting myocardial function and volume overload. Anemia in ACHD can occur as the result of pregnancy or menorrhagia, gastrointestinal blood loss, recent surgery or intervention, hemolysis caused by prosthetic valves, intracardiac patches or endocarditis, spontaneous bleeding from arteriovenous fistulas in the gut or lungs, hemoptysis in patients with severe pulmonary hypertension, or the use of anticoagulants. Moreover, anemia can occur because of chronic renal failure or other chronic disease.

Anemia, as conventionally defined, is rarely encountered in cyanotic patients. Chronic hypoxia results in an increase in erythropoietin production and an isolated rise in the red blood cell count (secondary erythrocytosis) [100]. This is a compensatory mechanism aimed at augmenting the amount of oxygen delivered to the tissues in the presence of significant right-to-left shunting. Relative anemia (ie, an inadequate rise in hemoglobin levels despite chronic cyanosis) can occur as a result of iron deficiency and is often detrimental to these delicate patients [101]. Unfortunately, there is no accepted algorithm for the calculation of appropriate hemoglobin levels, although it generally is accepted that a patient with a resting oxygen saturation of less than 85% should have a hemoglobin concentration of at least 18 g/dL. The diagnosis of relative anemia remains intuitive, and serum ferritin and transferrin saturation should be monitored [101].

*Pulmonary function*

There are data to suggest that pulmonary function in ACHD is impaired and could affect exercise capacity. Subnormal forced vital capacity has been reported in patients with Ebstein's anomaly, tetralogy of Fallot, congenitally corrected (l-) transposition, Fontan operation, atrial repair of transposition, and atrial septal defects [37,102,103]. In the authors' experience, pulmonary function expressed as percent of %FEV1 and forced vital capacity (%FVC) was depressed significantly in patients who have ACHD. %FEV1 was a powerful predictor of exercise capacity in this population [44]. Possible mechanisms for the abnormal pulmonary function observed in patients who have ACHD include prior surgery with lung scarring, atelectasis, chest deformities, diaphragmatic palsy, pulmonary vascular disease with loss of distensibility of peripheral arteries, significant cardiomegaly, and reduced blood supply to portions of the lung that become hypoplastic such as in the case of scimitar syndrome and pulmonary atresia.

*Endothelial dysfunction*

Endothelial dysfunction appears to play an important role in the pathophysiology of exercise intolerance in acquired heart failure [104,105]. It correlates to the degree of impairment and to brain natriuretic peptide levels. It is a predictor of outcome in patients with advanced heart failure and improves after heart failure treatment [45,106,107]. It is postulated that endothelial dysfunction has a detrimental effect on myocardial and skeletal muscle function. Evidence of endothelial dysfunction in CHD is available for pediatric patients after a Fontan-type operation and in those with Kawasaki disease [108–110]. In the Fontan group, endothelial function was related to exercise capacity, supporting the role of the endothelium in exercise adaptation [100]. Oechslin and colleagues recently provided evidence of systemic endothelial dysfunction and reduced basal nitric oxide availability in ACHD patients with cyanosis [111].

## Neurohormonal activation in adult congenital heart disease

Although cardiac dysfunction is the primary cause of the heart failure syndrome, the periphery plays a fundamental role in the pathophysiology of heart failure [112]. The reduction in blood flow to organs such as the kidney and the skeletal muscle appears to cause hyperactivation of the neuroendocrine system and of peripheral reflexes that control blood pressure and the ventilatory and chronotropic response to exertion. These, in turn, may be responsible for the onset of symptoms limiting exercise capacity and for perpetuating and aggravating heart failure itself. Modern heart failure treatment is based on agents such as angiotensin-converting enzyme inhibitors, beta adrenergic blockers, and aldosterone, which are aimed at reversing these changes.

Elevated levels of the atrial natriuretic peptide were first described in children with CHD by Lang and colleagues [113]. Thereafter, neurohormone levels were proposed as a means of assessing hemodynamic status, the adequacy of medical treatment, and the effect of surgery in such patients [114–116]. Bolger and colleagues described elevated levels of the natriuretic peptides, endothelin-1, norepinephrine, renin, and aldosterone in patients who had ACHD, even when asymptomatic [117]. Natriuretic peptides and endothelin levels were related to functional (NYHA) class, peak $VO_2$ and systemic ventricular function, and ECG and radiographic parameters. Activation of the natriuretic peptides occurs in a spectrum of congenital and noncongenital cardiac diseases and remains elevated for years after surgical repair of even relatively simple lesions [118]. Natriuretic peptide levels, therefore, appear to be a sensitive marker of cardiac dysfunction in ACHD and in acquired heart failure [119].

## Cytokine activation

Activation of cytokines also appears to play a role in the pathophysiology of heart failure, especially in advanced stages. Levine and colleagues showed that chronic heart failure is associated with cytokine activation [120]. Rauchhaus and colleagues extended this concept by demonstrating that raised inflammatory cytokine and cytokine receptor levels are strong prognostic markers in heart failure and seem to have direct toxic effects on the myocardium [121].

Sharma and colleagues reported high levels of cytokine expression in patients who have ACHD [122]. Tumor necrosis factor (TNF) levels correlated well to disease severity expressed as NYHA class. Patients with peripheral edema had significantly higher endotoxin levels, a potent stimulus for inflammatory cytokine production [123]. Cyanotic patients in particular were found to have significantly increased levels of inflammatory cytokines and a trend toward higher endotoxin levels [109]. Hypoxia is, in fact, a known trigger for inflammatory cytokine release in patients with heart failure [124]. Although TNF receptor (TNFR) concentrations in the serum were not significantly higher in patients compared with controls, a significant correlation was seen between levels of TNFR-1 and systemic ventricular function.

Similar studies on immune activation in CHD have focused on the pediatric population, especially in relation to surgery [125–127]. Lequier and colleagues noted that 40% of infants with congenital heart defects were significantly endotoxemic, with an adverse impact on clinical outcome [128]. Surgery, nevertheless, represents a strong stimulus for the production of inflammatory cytokines, and the results of these studies need to be interpreted with caution before making inferences to ACHD patients in general.

## Heart rate variability, baroreflex, and chemoreflex sensitivity

Deranged cardiac autonomic nervous activity is associated with adverse outcome in heart failure and coronary artery disease [129,130]. Heart rate variability and baroreflex sensitivity, both markers of cardiac autonomic nervous activity, are strong independent predictors of death after myocardial infarction and in chronic heart failure [106,131–133]. Evidence of autonomic dysfunction has been observed in ACHD [109,134,135]. Markedly deranged cardiac autonomic nervous control late after repair of tetralogy of Fallot and in patients after a Fontan-type operation has been reported by the authors' group [136,137]. Autonomic imbalance was related to the propensity for arrhythmias and to hemodynamic parameters such as the degree of pulmonary regurgitation, right ventricular end-systolic pressures, left and right ventricular ejection fractions, and QRS duration in patients with tetralogy of Fallot. Even though cardiac denervation secondary to surgery could play a role in cardiac autonomic derangement, a clear relationship between autonomic indices and hemodynamic status was present. The association of abnormal heart rate variability to both a history of arrhythmias and known markers of ventricular tachycardia and sudden cardiac death suggests a possible prognostic impact of autonomic parameters in ACHD.

Chemoreflex and peripheral metaboreflex (ergoreflex) hypersensitivity are recognized features of chronic heart failure and important predictors of reduced exercise tolerance and adverse prognosis [138,139]. Moreover, periodic breathing, characterized by oscillations in the depth of ventilation associated with oscillations in heart rate and blood pressure, is a powerful predictor of poor outcome in acquired heart failure [140]. Few data exist on the chemoreflex and ergoreflex sensitivity in ACHD. A small study by Brassard and colleagues reported that patients after a Fontan-type operation had excessive contribution of the ergoreflex to blood pressure but not to ventilatory variations. Moreover, Fontan patients had abnormal skeletal muscle function expressed as time to fatigue. After an 8-week training program, abnormal ergoreflex hyperactivation was reduced [141]. Georgiadou and colleagues reported two cases of periodic breathing and abnormal chemoreflex sensitivity in previously repaired tetralogy of Fallot [142].

## The prognostic value of parameters of exercise intolerance

Cardiopulmonary exercise testing is a useful tool for identifying patients at risk of hospitalization and death, and thus in need of particular attention and additional resources. Peak oxygen consumption and the $VE/VCO_2$ slope are established prognostic markers for the acquired heart failure population [1,2]. The authors' group reported that peak $VO_2$ was an independent predictor of outcome in the medium term (median follow-up 304 days) expressed as death or hospitalization [44]. Patients with a peak $VO_2$ less than 15.5 mL/kg/min demonstrated a 2.9-fold increased risk of hospital admission or death compared with patients with a peak $VO_2$ above 15.5 mL/kg/min. Moreover, peak $VO_2$ was related to the frequency and duration of hospitalization adjusted for follow-up time, even after accounting for NYHA class, age, age at surgery, and gender.

The $VE/VCO_2$ slope is also a strong predictor of outcome in ACHD and is stronger than peak $VO_2$ in predicting death in patients without cyanosis [16]. A $VE/VCO_2$ slope above 38 identified noncyanotic patients at higher risk of death in the mid-term. In the overall ACHD population, peak $VO_2$ remained the strongest independent predictor of outcome.

## Improving exercise tolerance in adult congenital heart disease

### Surgical and interventional options

Because cardiac dysfunction is a major determinant of exercise intolerance in ACHD, improved cardiac hemodynamics should be the first target in the effort to improve exercise capacity. Potential therapeutic options include surgical or interventional relief of obstructive lesions, repair of valve abnormalities, and closure of shunts. Improvement in symptoms has been reported after interventions such as Fontan-type operations, tetralogy of Fallot repair, relief of congenital aortic stenosis, and transcutaneous closure of ASD [143–147].

Resynchronization therapy has a role for treating patients who have left ventricular dysfunction and intraventricular conduction delay [148–150]. Preliminary studies of ventricular resynchronization in selected congenital cohorts have provided promising results. In biventricular hearts with significant intraventricular delay, Janousek and colleagues and Zimmerman and colleagues reported an increase in systolic blood pressure and cardiac index with biventricular pacing in the postoperative period [151,152]. Dubin and colleagues showed an acute increase in cardiac output and right ventricular systolic performance in patients who had intraventricular delay [153]. Recently, a multi-center registry reported the results of biventricular pacing on 103 pediatric patients, 73 of whom had CHD [154]. Overall, a significant increase in systemic ventricular ejection fraction and a decrease in QRS duration were observed. These findings were confirmed when patients with a systemic right ventricle were examined separately, but they were not found in the overall CHD group. In univentricular hearts, QRS duration decreased significantly, and a trend for an increase in ejection fraction was seen ($P = .08$), despite the small sample size. Thus, resynchronization therapy may benefit patients who have CHD. Further, prospective studies are needed to establish the beneficial effects of biventricular pacing in ACHD and to identify patients who are more likely to benefit from resynchronization therapy.

**Medical management**

Neurohormonal blockade is the cornerstone of modern chronic heart failure treatment. Angiotensin-converting enzyme inhibitors (ACEi), angiotensin receptor antagonists, spironolactone, and beta blockers not only improve hemodynamics but also slow the progression of heart failure and improve prognosis. Unfortunately, only limited data are available on the use of ACEi and beta blockers for improving exercise tolerance in the congenital population [155]. ACEi are often used empirically, especially in cases of right and left ventricular volume overload [156–160]. The evidence for the use of beta blockers is even scantier [161–164].

Recently, numerous drugs have become available for treating primary pulmonary hypertension, some of which may be applicable to ACHD patients who have pulmonary arterial hypertension. Fernadez and colleagues recently demonstrated that epoprostenol improves functional capacity, systemic saturations, and pulmonary hemodynamics in patients who have CHD and pulmonary arterial hypertension [165]. The use of epoprostenol is, however, limited by its invasive nature and associated complications such as line and systemic infections and line dislocations. Sildenafil, an oral phospodiasterase-5-inhibitor, has been shown to improve functional capacity in patients who have pulmonary arterial hypertension, including some with CHD [166]. Bosentan, an oral dual receptor endothelin antagonist, has been demonstrated to improve exercise capacity in patients with Eisenmenger syndrome, both in several open-label intention-to-treat pilot studies, and in a recently reported randomized placebo-controlled study [167–171]. Although long-term data are lacking, Bosentan appears to be the most promising treatment for highly symptomatic ACHD patients who have significant pulmonary arterial hypertension.

**Exercise training and recommendations for exercise**

The psychological and physical benefits of exercise training on patients who have acquired heart disease are well-established [172]; however, limited data exist on the effect of exercise training in patients who have ACHD. Systematic training programs have only been introduced to small cohorts of ACHD patients, and most studies conclude that the exercise training is safe and might be beneficial, although no significant effect on exercise capacity has been demonstrated [173,174].

It is generally accepted that physical exercise of appropriate intensity should be encouraged in most patients who have ACHD. Recommendations for the participation of patients with CHD in sports according to the underlying anatomy and physiology were issued after the 36th Bethesda Conference [175]. Counseling should, nevertheless, also include an estimation of the type of exercise and its potential impact on cardiac hemodynamics [176]. Exercise testing can be invaluable in aiding clinical judgment, as it reproduces the conditions of stress during sports activities under electrocardiographic and blood pressure monitoring. High-impact sport is best avoided in patients with Marfan's syndrome or other aortic anomalies and those on anticoagulation therapy or carrying a pacemaker. Particular attention should be paid to patients at high risk of arrhythmia and sudden death, such as those with arrhythmogenic right ventricular dysplasia, hypertrophic obstructive cardiomyopathy and long QT syndrome. Recommendations should be discussed with patients, and simple preventive measures such avoiding excessive dehydration should be suggested.

**Is exercise intolerance in adult congenital heart disease heart failure?**

It is clear that important similarities exist between ACHD and heart failure syndrome [177]. Current heart failure management is evidence-based, modeled on the results of large randomized controlled trials with hard end points such as death. Such evidence is difficult to acquire in a relatively small and heterogeneous population such as that of ACHD patients, with a relatively low overall annual mortality rate. Despite the lack of evidence, heart failure medication such as ACE inhibitors is used widely in ACHD. An effort should be made to gather data on the potential beneficial effects of established heart failure therapies through the creation of a network of ACHD centers and the design of registries and multi-center studies. Conversely, investigations of the pathophysiology of exercise intolerance in

ACHD could provide interesting insights for understanding exercise limitation in acquired heart failure.

## Summary

Exercise intolerance is prevalent in the ACHD population and affects patients from all diagnostic groups, including those with simple lesions. Cardiopulmonary exercise testing, with the calculation of peak $VO_2$ and the $VE/VCO_2$ slope, provides a reliable tool for assessing the exercise capacity of ACHD patients and for risk stratification. This should become part of the routine clinical assessment of these patients. The relief of hemodynamic burdens and reconditioning through exercise training appear to be the management of choice. Moreover, similarities in the pathophysiology of exercise intolerance in acquired heart failure and CHD suggest that established heart failure therapies might be beneficial to ACHD patients with exercise intolerance, but their safety and efficacy should be established by multi-center randomized controlled trials.

## References

[1] Engelfriet P, Boersma E, Oechslin E, et al. The spectrum of adult congenital heart disease in Europe: morbidity and mortality in a 5 year follow-up period. The Euro Heart Survey on adult congenital heart disease. Eur Heart J 2005;26(21): 2325–33.

[2] Culbert EL, Ashburn DA, Cullen-Dean G, et al. Quality of life of children after repair of transposition of the great arteries. Circulation 2003;108: 857–62.

[3] Kamphuis M, Ottenkamp J, Vliegen HW, et al. Health-related quality of life and health status in adult survivors with previously operated complex congenital heart disease. Heart 2002;87:356–62.

[4] Moons P, Van Deyk K, Budts W, et al. Caliber of quality-of-life assessments in congenital heart disease: a plea for more conceptual and methodological rigor. Arch Pediatr Adolesc Med 2004;158(11): 1062–9.

[5] Hunt SA. American College of Cardiology. ACC/AHA 2005 guideline update for the diagnosis and management of chronic heart failure in the adult: a report of the American College of Cardiology/American Heart Association Task Force on Practice Guidelines (Writing Committee to Update the 2001 Guidelines for the Evaluation and Management of Heart Failure). J Am Coll Cardiol 2005; 46(6):e1–82.

[6] Swedberg K, Cleland J, Dargie H, et al. Guidelines for the diagnosis and treatment of chronic heart failure: executive summary (update 2005): the Task Force for the Diagnosis and Treatment of Chronic Heart Failure of the European Society of Cardiology. Eur Heart J 2005;26(11):1115–40.

[7] Bolger AP, Gatzoulis MA. Towards defining heart failure in adults with congenital heart disease. Int J Cardiol 2004;97(Suppl 1):15–23.

[8] Kamphuis M, Zwinderman KH, Vogels T, et al. A cardiac-specific health-related quality of life module for young adults with congenital heart disease: development and validation. Qual Life Res 2004; 13(4):735–45.

[9] Wasserman K, Hansen J, Sue D, Whipp B. Exercise testing and Interpretation: an overview. In: Principles of exercise testing and interpretation. Baltimore (MD): Lippincott Williams and Wilkins; 1999. p. 1–9.

[10] Cooper CB, Storer TW. Purpose. In: Exercise testing and interpretation. Cambridge (UK): Cambridge University Press; 2001. p. 1–14.

[11] Wasserman K, Hansen J, Sue D, et al. Measurements during integrative cardiopulmonary exercise testing. In: Principles of exercise testing and interpretation. Baltimore (MD): Lippincott Williams and Wilkins; 1999. p. 62–94.

[12] Cooper CB, Storer TW. Response variables. In: Exercise testing and interpretation. Cambridge (UK): Cambridge University Press; 2001. p. 93–148.

[13] Task Force of the Italian Working Group on Cardiac Rehabilitation Prevention. Statement on cardiopulmonary exercise testing in chronic heart failure due to left ventricular dysfunction: recommendations for performance and interpretation Part I: definition of cardiopulmonary exercise testing parameters for appropriate use in chronic heart failure. Eur J Cardiovasc Prev Rehabil 2006;13(2): 150–64.

[14] Gitt AK, Wasserman K, Kilkowski C, et al. Exercise anaerobic threshold and ventilatory efficiency identify heart failure patients for high risk of early death. Circulation 2002;106:3079–84.

[15] Francis DP, Shamim W, Davies LC, et al. Cardiopulmonary exercise testing for prognosis in chronic heart failure: continuous and independent prognostic value from $VE/VCO_2$ slope and peak VO2. Eur Heart J 2000;21(2):154–61.

[16] Dimopoulos K, Okonko DO, Diller GP, et al. Abnormal ventilatory response to exercise in adults with congenital heart disease relates to cyanosis and predicts survival. Circulation 2006;113: 2796–802.

[17] Ponikowski P, Francis DP, Piepoli MF, et al. Enhanced ventilatory response to exercise in patients with chronic heart failure and preserved exercise tolerance: marker of abnormal cardiorespiratory reflex control and predictor of poor prognosis. Circulation 2001;103:967–72.

[18] Chua TP, Ponikowski P, Harrington D, et al. Clinical correlates and prognostic significance of the

ventilatory response to exercise in chronic heart failure. J Am Coll Cardiol 1997;29(7):1585–90.

[19] Tabet JY, Beauvais F, Thabut G, et al. A critical appraisal of the prognostic value of the $VE/VCO_2$ slope in chronic heart failure. Eur J Cardiovasc Prev Rehabil 2003;10:267–72.

[20] Cooper CB, Storer TW. Testing methods. In: Exercise testing and interpretation. Cambridge (UK): Cambridge University Press; 2001. p. 51–92.

[21] Niedeggen A, Skobel E, Haager P, et al. Comparison of the 6-minute walk test with established parameters for assessment of cardiopulmonary capacity in adults with complex congenital cardiac disease. Cardiol Young 2005;15(4):385–90.

[22] Hoeper MM, Oudiz RJ, Peacock A, et al. End points and clinical trial designs in pulmonary arterial hypertension: clinical and regulatory perspectives. J Am Coll Cardiol 2004;43:48S–55S.

[23] ATS Committee on Proficiency Standards for Clinical Pulmonary Function Laboratories. ATS statement: guidelines for the six-minute walk test. Am J Respir Crit Care Med 2002;166:111–7.

[24] Oudiz RJ, Barst RJ, Hansen JE, et al. Cardiopulmonary exercise testing and six-minute walk correlations in pulmonary arterial hypertension. Am J Cardiol 2006;97(1):123–6.

[25] Frost AE, Langleben D, Oudiz R, et al. The 6-min walk test (6MW) as an efficacy end point in pulmonary arterial hypertension clinical trials: demonstration of a ceiling effect. Vascul Pharmacol 2005;43(1):36–9.

[26] Wu G, Sanderson B, Bittner V. The 6-minute walk test: how important is the learning effect? Am Heart J 2003;146(1):129–33.

[27] Veldtman GR, Nishimoto A, Siu S, et al. The Fontan procedure in adults. Heart 2001;86(3):330–5.

[28] Alphonso N, Baghai M, Sundar P, et al. Intermediate-term outcome following the Fontan operation: a survival, functional and risk-factor analysis. Eur J Cardiothorac Surg 2005;28(4):529–35.

[29] Daliento L, Somerville J, Presbitero P, et al. Eisenmenger syndrome. Factors relating to deterioration and death. Eur Heart J 1998;19:1845–55.

[30] Graham TP Jr, Bernard YD, Mellen BG, et al. Long-term outcome in congenitally corrected transposition of the great arteries: a multi-institutional study. J Am Coll Cardiol 2000;36:255–61.

[31] Beauchesne LM, Warnes CA, Connolly HM, et al. Outcome of the unoperated adult who presents with congenitally corrected transposition of the great arteries. J Am Coll Cardiol 2002;40:285–90.

[32] Piran S, Veldtman G, Siu S, et al. Heart failure and ventricular dysfunction in patients with single or systemic right ventricles. Circulation 2002;105(10):1189–94.

[33] Norozi K, Buchhorn R, Kaiser C, et al. Plasma N-terminal probrain natriuretic peptide as a marker of right ventricular dysfunction in patients with tetralogy of Fallot after surgical repair. Chest 2005;128(4):2563–70.

[34] de Ruijter FT, Weenink I, Hitchcock F, et al. Right ventricular dysfunction and pulmonary valve replacement after correction of tetralogy of Fallot. Ann Thorac Surg 2002;73:1794–800.

[35] Sietsema KE, Cooper DM, Perloff JK, et al. Dynamics of oxygen uptake during exercise in adults with cyanotic congenital heart disease. Circulation 1986;73:1137–44.

[36] Clark AL, Swan JW, Laney R, et al. The role of right and left ventricular function in the ventilatory response to exercise in chronic heart failure. Circulation 1994;89:2062–9.

[37] Fredriksen PM, Veldtman G, Hechter S, et al. Aerobic capacity in adults with various congenital heart diseases. Am J Cardiol 2001;87:310–4.

[38] Hechter SJ, Webb G, Fredriksen PM, et al. Cardiopulmonary exercise performance in adult survivors of the Mustard procedure. Cardiol Young 2001;11:407–14.

[39] Fredriksen PM, Chen A, Veldtman G, et al. Exercise capacity in adult patients with congenitally corrected transposition of the great arteries. Heart 2001;85:191–5.

[40] Glaser S, Opitz CF, Bauer U, et al. Assessment of symptoms and exercise capacity in cyanotic patients with congenital heart disease. Chest 2004;125(2):368–76.

[41] Harrison DA, Liu P, Walters JE, et al. Cardiopulmonary function in adult patients late after Fontan repair. J Am Coll Cardiol 1995;26:1016–21.

[42] Fredriksen PM, Veldtman G, Hechter S, et al. Aerobic capacity in adults with various congenital heart diseases. Am J Cardiol 2001;87:310–4.

[43] Fredriksen PM, Therrien J, Veldtman G, et al. Aerobic capacity in adults with tetralogy of Fallot. Cardiol Young 2002;12:554–9.

[44] Diller GP, Dimopoulos K, Okonko D, et al. Exercise intolerance in adult congenital heart disease: comparative severity, correlates, and prognostic implication. Circulation 2005;112(6):828–35.

[45] Clark AL, Poole-Wilson PA, Coats AJ. Exercise limitation in chronic heart failure: central role of the periphery. J Am Coll Cardiol 1996;28(5):1092–102.

[46] Lipkin DP, Poole-Wilson PA. Symptoms limiting exercise in chronic heart failure. Br Med J (Clin Res Ed) 1986;292(6527):1030–1.

[47] Reybrouck T, Boshoff D, Vanhees L, et al. Ventilatory response to exercise in patients after correction of cyanotic congenital heart disease: relation with clinical outcome after surgery. Heart 2004;90:215–6.

[48] Wasserman K, Stringer WW, Sun XG, et al. Circulatory coupling of external to muscler respiration during exercise. In: Wasserman K, editor. Cardiopulmonary exercise testing and cardiovascular

health. Armonk (NY): Futura Publishing Company; 2002. p. 3–26.

[49] Takagaki M, Ishino K, Kawada M, et al. Total right ventricular exclusion improves left ventricular function in patients with end-stage congestive right ventricular failure. Circulation 2003;108:II226–9.

[50] Davlouros PA, Kilner PJ, Hornung TS, et al. Right ventricular function in adults with repaired tetralogy of Fallot assessed with cardiovascular magnetic resonance imaging: detrimental role of right ventricular outflow aneurysms or akinesia and adverse right-to-left ventricular interaction. J Am Coll Cardiol 2002;40:2044–52.

[51] Hurwitz RA, Caldwell RL, Girod DA, et al. Right ventricular systolic function in adolescents and young adults after Mustard operation for transposition of the great arteries. Am J Cardiol 1996;77: 294–7.

[52] Hornung TS, Kilner PJ, Davlouros PA, et al. Excessive right ventricular hypertrophic response in adults with the Mustard procedure for transposition of the great arteries. Am J Cardiol 2002;90: 800–3.

[53] Lubiszewska B, Gosiewska E, Hoffman P, et al. Myocardial perfusion and function of the systemic right ventricle in patients after atrial switch procedure for complete transposition: long-term follow-up. J Am Coll Cardiol 2000;36(4):1365–70.

[54] Dodge-Khatami A, Tulevski II, Bennink GB, et al. Comparable systemic ventricular function in healthy adults and patients with unoperated congenitally corrected transposition using MRI dobutamine stress testing. Ann Thorac Surg 2002;73: 1759–64.

[55] Tulevski II, Zijta FM, Smeijers AS, et al. Regional and global right ventricular dysfunction in asymptomatic or minimally symptomatic patients with congenitally corrected transposition. Cardiol Young 2004;14(2):168–73.

[56] Hornung TS, Bernard EJ, Celermajer DS, et al. Right ventricular dysfunction in congenitally corrected transposition of the great arteries. Am J Cardiol 1999;84:1116–9.

[57] Millane T, Bernard EJ, Jaeggi E, et al. Role of ischemia and infarction in late right ventricular dysfunction after atrial repair of transposition of the great arteries. J Am Coll Cardiol 2000;35: 1661–8.

[58] Davlouros PA, Niwa K, Webb G, et al. The right ventricle in congenital heart disease. Heart 2006; 92(Suppl 1):i27–38.

[59] Yoerger DM, Marcus F, Sherrill D, et al. Echocardiographic findings in patients meeting task force criteria for arrhythmogenic right ventricular dysplasia: new insights from the multidisciplinary study of right ventricular dysplasia. J Am Coll Cardiol 2005;45(6):860–5.

[60] Allen BS, Winkelmann JW, Hanafy H, et al. Retrograde cardioplegia does not adequately perfuse the right ventricle. J Thorac Cardiovasc Surg 1995; 109(6):1116–24.

[61] Li W, Somerville J, Gibson DG, et al. Effect of atrial flutter on exercise tolerance in patients with grown-up congenital heart (GUCH). Am Heart J 2002;144:173–9.

[62] Katritsis D, Camm AJ. Chronotropic incompetence: a proposal for definition and diagnosis. Br Heart J 1993;70:400–2.

[63] Astrand A. Aerobic work capacity in men and women with special reference to age. Acta Physiol Scand 1960;49:1–92.

[64] Witte KK, Cleland JG, Clark AL. Chronic heart failure, chronotropic incompetence, and the effects of beta blockade. Heart 2006;92:481–6.

[65] Lauer MS, Okin PM, Larson MG, et al. Impaired heart rate response to graded exercise. Prognostic implications of chronotropic incompetence in the Framingham Heart Study. Circulation 1996;93: 1520–6.

[66] Lauer MS, Francis GS, Okin PM, et al. Impaired chronotropic response to exercise stress testing as a predictor of mortality. JAMA 1999;281:524–9.

[67] Jouven X, Empana JP, Schwartz PJ, et al. Heart-rate profile during exercise as a predictor of sudden death. N Engl J Med 2005;352:1951–8.

[68] Fredriksen PM, Ingjer F, Nystad W, et al. A comparison of $VO_2$ (peak) between patients with congenital heart disease and healthy subjects, all aged 8–17 years. Eur J Appl Physiol Occup Physiol 1999;80(5):409–16.

[69] Diller GP, Okonko DO, von Haehling S, et al. Chronotropic incompetence in adult patients with systemic right ventricle and univentricular circulation. J Am Coll Cardiol 2005;45:325A.

[70] Diller GP, Dimopoulos K, Okonko DO, et al. Heart rate response during exercise and recovery is an independent predictor of death in adult congenital heart disease patients. Available at: http://www.abstractsonline.com/arch/RecordView.aspx?LookupKey=12345&recordID=18423. Accessed March 18, 2006.

[71] Colucci WS, Ribeiro JR, Rocco MB, et al. Impaired chronotropic response to exercise in patients with congestive heart failure. Role of postsynaptic beta-adrenergic desensitization. Circulation 1989; 80:314–23.

[72] Fei L, Keeling PJ, Sadoul N, et al. Decreased heart rate variability in patients with congestive heart failure and chronotropic incompetence. Pacing Clin Electrophysiol 1996;19:477–83.

[73] Paul T, Blaufox AD, Saul JP. Invasive electrophysiology and pacing. In: Gatzoulis MA, Webb GD, Daubeney PE, editors. Diagnosis and management of adult congenital heart disease. London: Churchill Livingstone; 2003. p. 115–24.

[74] O'Keefe JH Jr, Abuissa H, Jones PG, et al. Effect of chronic right ventricular apical pacing on left ventricular function. Am J Cardiol 2005;95:771–3.

[75] Nielsen JC, Kristensen L, Andersen HR, et al. A randomized comparison of atrial and dual chamber pacing in 177 consecutive patients with sick sinus syndrome: echocardiographic and clinical outcome. J Am Coll Cardiol 2003;42:614–23.

[76] Thambo JB, Bordachar P, Garrigue S, et al. Detrimental ventricular remodeling in patients with congenital complete heart block and chronic right ventricular apical pacing. Circulation 2004; 110(25):3766–72.

[77] Rinfret S, Cohen DJ, Lamas GA, et al. Cost-effectiveness of dual-chamber pacing compared with ventricular pacing for sinus node dysfunction. Circulation 2005;111(2):165–72.

[78] Selden R, Schaefer RA, Kennedy BJ, et al. Corrected transposition of the great arteries simulating coronary heart disease in adults. Chest 1976;69(2): 188–91.

[79] Weindling SN, Wernovsky G, Colan SD, et al. Myocardial perfusion, function and exercise tolerance after the arterial switch operation. J Am Coll Cardiol 1994;23:424–33.

[80] Hayes AM, Baker EJ, Kakadeker A, et al. Influence of anatomic correction for transposition of the great arteries on myocardial perfusion: radionuclide imaging with technetium–99m 2–methoxy isobutyl isonitrile. J Am Coll Cardiol 1994;24: 769–77.

[81] Bengel FM, Hauser M, Duvernoy CS, et al. Myocardial blood flow and coronary flow reserve late after anatomical correction of transposition of the great arteries. J Am Coll Cardiol 1998; 32(7):1955–61.

[82] Babu-Narayan SV, Kilner PJ, Li W, et al. Ventricular fibrosis suggested by cardiovascular magnetic resonance in adults with repaired tetralogy of Fallot and its relationship to adverse markers of clinical outcome. Circulation 2006;113(3):405–13.

[83] Babu-Narayan SV, Goktekin O, Moon JC, et al. Late gadolinium enhancement cardiovascular magnetic resonance of the systemic right ventricle in adults with previous atrial redirection surgery for transposition of the great arteries. Circulation 2005;111(16):2091–8.

[84] Senzaki H, Masutani S, Kobayashi J, et al. Ventricular afterload and ventricular work in Fontan circulation: comparison with normal two-ventricle circulation and single-ventricle circulation with Blalock-Taussig shunts. Circulation 2002;105: 2885–92.

[85] Singh TP, Humes RA, Muzik O, et al. Myocardial flow reserve in patients with a systemic right ventricle after atrial switch repair. J Am Coll Cardiol 2001;37(8):2120–5.

[86] Hauser M, Bengel FM, Kuhn A, et al. Myocardial perfusion and coronary flow reserve assessed by positron emission tomography in patients after Fontan-like operations. Pediatr Cardiol 2003; 24(4):386–92.

[87] Meijboom FJ. Constrictive pericarditis and restrictive cardiomyopathy. In: Gatzoulis MA, Webb GD, Daubeney PE, editors. Diagnosis and management of adult congenital heart disease. London: Churchill Livingstone; 2003. p. 459–66.

[88] Gatzoulis MA, Munk MD, Merchant N, et al. Isolated congenital absence of the pericardium: clinical presentation, diagnosis, and management. Ann Thorac Surg 2000;69(4):1209–15.

[89] Abbas AE, Appleton CP, Liu PT, et al. Congenital absence of the pericardium: case presentation and review of literature. Int J Cardiol 2005;98(1):21–5.

[90] Rheuban KS. Pericardial diseases. In: Allen HD, Gutgesell HP, Clark EB, editors. Heart disease in infants, children and adolescents. 6th edition. Philadelphia: Lippincott Williams and Wilkins; 2001. p. 1287–97.

[91] van Son JA, Danielson GK, Callahan JA. Congenital absence of the pericardium: displacement of the heart associated with tricuspid insufficiency. Ann Thorac Surg 1993;56(6):1405–6.

[92] Chatzis AC, Giannopoulos NM, Sarris GE. Isolated congenital tricuspid insufficiency associated with right-sided congenital partial absence of the pericardium. J Heart Valve Dis 2004;13(5):790–1.

[93] Goetz WA, Liebold A, Vogt F, et al. Tricuspid valve repair in a case with congenital absence of left thoracic pericardium. Eur J Cardiothorac Surg 2004;26(4):848–9.

[94] Fukuda N, Oki T, Iuchi A, et al. Pulmonary and systemic venous flow patterns assessed by transesophageal Doppler echocardiography in congenital absence of the pericardium. Am J Cardiol 1995; 75(17):1286–8.

[95] Oki T, Tabata T, Yamada H, et al. Cross sectional echocardiographic demonstration of the mechanisms of abnormal interventricular septal motion in congenital total absence of the left pericardium. Heart 1997;77(3):247–51.

[96] Harris L, Belaji S. Arrhythmias in the adult with congenital heart disease. In: Gatzoulis MA, Webb GD, Daubeney PE, editors. Diagnosis and management of adult congenital heart disease. London: Churchill Livingstone; 2003. p. 105–13.

[97] Sietsema KE, Cooper DM, Perloff JK, et al. Control of ventilation during exercise in patients with central venous-to-systemic arterial shunts. J Appl Physiol 1988;64(1):234–42.

[98] Oudiz RJ, Sun XG. Abnormalities in exercise gas exchange in primary pulmonary hypertension. In: Wasserman K, editor: Cardiopulmonary exercise testing and cardiovascular health. Futura, Armonk (NY): 2002. p. 179–90.

[99] Sun XG, Hansen JE, Oudiz RJ, et al. Exercise pathophysiology in patients with primary pulmonary hypertension. Circulation 2001;104(4):429–35.

[100] Oechslin E. Eisenmenger's syndrome. In: Gatzoulis MA, Webb GD, Daubeney PE, editors. Diagnosis and management of adult congenital

heart disease. London: Churchill Livingstone; 2003. p. 363–77.

[101] Broberg CS, Bax BE, Okonko DO, et al. Blood viscosity and its relation to iron deficiency, symptoms, and exercise capacity in adults with cyanotic congenital heart disease. J Am Coll Cardiol 2006;48: 356–65.

[102] Fredriksen PM, Therrien J, Veldtman G, et al. Lung function and aerobic capacity in adult patients following modified Fontan procedure. Heart 2001;85(3):295–9.

[103] Sulc J, Andrle V, Hruda J, et al. Pulmonary function in children with atrial septal defect before and after heart surgery. Heart 1998;80(5):484–8.

[104] Bank A, Lee P, Kubo S. Endothelial dysfunction in patients with heart failure: relationship to disease severity. J Card Fail 2000;6(1):29–36.

[105] Lerman A, Zeiher AM. Endothelial function: cardiac events. Circulation 2005;111(3):363–8.

[106] Katz SD, Hryniewicz K, Hriljac I, et al. Vascular endothelial dysfunction and mortality risk in patients with chronic heart failure. Circulation 2005; 111:310–4.

[107] Fischer D, Rossa S, Landmesser U, et al. Endothelial dysfunction in patients with chronic heart failure is independently associated with increased incidence of hospitalization, cardiac transplantation, or death. Eur Heart J 2005;26(1):65–9.

[108] Mahle WT, Todd K, Fyfe DA. Endothelial function following the Fontan operation. Am J Cardiol 2003;91(10):1286–8.

[109] Dhillon R, Clarkson P, Donald AE, et al. Endothelial dysfunction late after Kawasaki disease. Circulation 1996;94(9):2103–6.

[110] Deng YB, Li TL, Xiang HJ, et al. Impaired endothelial function in the brachial artery after Kawasaki disease and the effects of intravenous administration of vitamin C. Pediatr Infect Dis J 2003;22(1):34–9.

[111] Oechslin E, Kiowski W, Schindler R, et al. Systemic endothelial dysfunction in adults with cyanotic congenital heart disease. Circulation 2005;112(8): 1106–12.

[112] Coats AJ. The muscle hypothesis of chronic heart failure. J Mol Cell Cardiol 1996;28(11):2255–62.

[113] Lang RE, Unger T, Ganten D, et al. Alpha atrial natriuretic peptide concentrations in plasma of children with congenital heart and pulmonary diseases. Br Med J (Clin Res Ed) 1985;291:1241.

[114] Kikuchi K, Nishioka K, Ueda T, et al. Relationship between plasma atrial natriuretic polypeptide concentration and hemodynamic measurements in children with congenital heart diseases. J Pediatr 1987;111:335–42.

[115] Ross RD, Daniels SR, Schwartz DC, et al. Return of plasma norepinephrine to normal after resolution of congestive heart failure in congenital heart disease. Am J Cardiol 1987;60:1411–3.

[116] Ishikawa S, Miyauchi T, Sakai S, et al. Elevated levels of plasma endothelin-1 in young patients with pulmonary hypertension caused by congenital heart disease are decreased after successful surgical repair. J Thorac Cardiovasc Surg 1995; 110:271–3.

[117] Genth-Zotz S, von Haehling S, Bolger AP, et al. Neurohormonal activation and the chronic heart failure syndrome in adults with congenital heart disease. Circulation 2002;106:92–9.

[118] Iivainen TE, Groundstroem KW, Lahtela JT, et al. Serum N-terminal atrial natriuretic peptide in adult patients late after surgical repair of atrial septal defect. Eur J Heart Fail 2000;2:161–5.

[119] Tulevski II, Groenink M, van Der Wall EE, et al. Increased brain and atrial natriuretic peptides in patients with chronic right ventricular pressure overload: correlation between plasma neurohormones and right ventricular dysfunction. Heart 2001;86:27–30.

[120] Levine B, Kalman J, Mayer L, et al. Elevated circulating levels of tumor necrosis factor in severe chronic heart failure. N Engl J Med 1990;323(4): 236–41.

[121] Rauchhaus M, Doehner W, Francis DP, et al. Plasma cytokine parameters and mortality in patients with chronic heart failure. Circulation 2000; 102(25):3060–7.

[122] Sharma R, Bolger AP, Li W, et al. Elevated circulating levels of inflammatory cytokines and bacterial endotoxin in adults with congenital heart disease. Am J Cardiol 2003;92(2):188–93.

[123] Niebauer J, Volk HD, Kemp M, et al. Endotoxin and immune activation in chronic heart failure: a prospective cohort study. Lancet 1999; 353(9167):1838–42.

[124] Hasper D, Hummel M, Kleber FX, et al. Systemic inflammation in patients with heart failure. Eur Heart J 1998;19:761–5.

[125] Ashraf SS, Tian Y, Zacharrias S, et al. Effects of cardiopulmonary bypass on neonatal and pediatric inflammatory profiles. Eur J Cardiothorac Surg 1997;12:862–8.

[126] Seghaye M, Duchateau J, Bruniaux J, et al. Interleukin-10 release related to cardiopulmonary bypass in infants undergoing cardiac operations. J Thorac Cardiovasc Surg 1996;111:545–53.

[127] Casey WF, Hauser GJ, Hannallah RS, et al. Circulating endotoxin and tumor necrosis factor during pediatric cardiac surgery. Crit Care Med 1992;20: 1090–6.

[128] Lequier LL, Nikaidoh H, Leonard SR, et al. Preoperative and postoperative endotoxemia in children with congenital heart disease. Chest 2000;117: 1706–12.

[129] Zipes DP, Levy MN, Cobb LA, et al. Sudden cardiac death. Neural-cardiac interactions. Circulation 1987;76:I202–7.

[130] Schwartz PJ. The autonomic nervous system and sudden death. Eur Heart J 1998;19(Suppl F): F72–80.

[131] Kleiger RE, Miller JP, Bigger JT Jr, et al. Decreased heart rate variability and its association with increased mortality after acute myocardial infarction. Am J Cardiol 1987;59:256–62.

[132] La Rovere MT, Bigger JT Jr, Marcus FI, et al. Baroreflex sensitivity and heart-rate variability in prediction of total cardiac mortality after myocardial infarction. ATRAMI (Autonomic Tone and Reflexes After Myocardial Infarction) Investigators. Lancet 1998;351:478–84.

[133] Ponikowski P, Anker SD, Chua TP, et al. Depressed heart rate variability as an independent predictor of death in chronic congestive heart failure secondary to ischemic or idiopathic dilated cardiomyopathy. Am J Cardiol 1997;79:1645–50.

[134] McLeod KA, Hillis WS, Houston AB, et al. Reduced heart rate variability following repair of tetralogy of Fallot. Heart 1999;81:656–60.

[135] Folino AF, Russo G, Bauce B, et al. Autonomic profile and arrhythmic risk stratification after surgical repair of tetralogy of Fallot. Am Heart J 2004;148(6):985–9.

[136] Davos CH, Francis DP, Leenarts MF, et al. Global impairment of cardiac autonomic nervous activity late after the Fontan operation. Circulation 2003; 108(Suppl 1):II180–5.

[137] Davos CH, Davlouros PA, Wensel R, et al. Global impairment of cardiac autonomic nervous activity late after repair of tetralogy of Fallot. Circulation 2002;106:I69–75.

[138] Piepoli M, Clark AL, Volterrani M, et al. Contribution of muscle afferents to the hemodynamic, autonomic, and ventilatory responses to exercise in patients with chronic heart failure: effects of physical training. Circulation 1996;93(5):940–52.

[139] Ponikowski P, Chua TP, Anker SD, et al. Peripheral chemoreceptor hypersensitivity: an ominous sign in patients with chronic heart failure. Circulation 2001;104(5):544–9.

[140] Francis DP, Willson K, Davies LC, et al. Quantitative general theory of periodic breathing in chronic heart failure and its clinical implications. Circulation 2000;102:2214–21.

[141] Brassard P, Poirier P, Martin J, et al. Impact of exercise training on muscle function and ergoreflex in Fontan patients: a pilot study. Int J Cardiol 2006; 107(1):85–94.

[142] Georgiadou P, Babu-Narayan SV, Francis DP, et al. Periodic breathing as a feature of right heart failure in congenital heart disease. Heart 2004; 90(9):1075–6.

[143] Mott AR, Feltes TF, McKenzie ED, et al. Improved early results with the Fontan operation in adults with functional single ventricle. Ann Thorac Surg 2004;77(4):1334–40.

[144] Borowski A, Ghodsizad A, Litmathe J, et al. Severe pulmonary regurgitation late after total repair of tetralogy of Fallot: surgical considerations. Pediatr Cardiol 2004;25(5):466–71.

[145] Brown JW, Ruzmetov M, Vijay P, et al. Surgical repair of congenital supravalvular aortic stenosis in children. Eur J Cardiothorac Surg 2002;21(1):50–6.

[146] Masetti P, Ussia GP, Gazzolo D, et al. Aortic pulmonary autograft implant: medium-term follow-up with a note on a new right ventricular pulmonary artery conduit. J Card Surg 1998;13(3):173–6.

[147] Brochu MC, Baril JF, Dore A, et al. Improvement in exercise capacity in asymptomatic and mildly symptomatic adults after atrial septal defect percutaneous closure. Circulation 2002;106(14):1821–6.

[148] Bristow MR, Saxon LA, Boehmer J, et al. Cardiac-resynchronization therapy with or without an implantable defibrillator in advanced chronic heart failure. N Engl J Med 2004;350:2140–50.

[149] Young JB, Abraham WT, Smith AL, et al. Combined cardiac resynchronization and implantable cardioversion defibrillation in advanced chronic heart failure: the MIRACLE ICD trial. JAMA 2003;289:2685–94.

[150] Cazeau S, Leclercq C, Lavergne T, et al. Effects of multi-site biventricular pacing in patients with heart failure and intraventricular conduction delay. N Engl J Med 2001;344:873–80.

[151] Janousek J, Vojtovic P, Hucin B, et al. Resynchronization pacing is a useful adjunct to the management of acute heart failure after surgery for congenital heart defects. Am J Cardiol 2001;88: 145–52.

[152] Zimmerman FJ, Starr JP, Koenig PR, et al. Acute hemodynamic benefit of multisite ventricular pacing after congenital heart surgery. Ann Thorac Surg 2003;75:1775–80.

[153] Dubin AM, Feinstein JA, Reddy VM, et al. Electrical resynchronization: a novel therapy for the failing right ventricle. Circulation 2003;107:2287–9.

[154] Dubin AM, Janousek J, Rhee E, et al. Resynchronization therapy in pediatric and congenital heart disease patients: an international multicenter study. J Am Coll Cardiol 2005;46(12):2277–83.

[155] Vonder Muhll I, Liu P, Webb G. Applying standard therapies to new targets: the use of ACE inhibitors and B-blockers for heart failure in adults with congenital heart disease. Int J Cardiol 2004; 97(Suppl 1):25–33.

[156] Alehan D, Ozkutlu S. Beneficial effects of 1-year captopril therapy in children with chronic aortic regurgitation who have no symptoms. Am Heart J 1998;135:598–603.

[157] Mori Y, Nakazawa M, Tomimatsu H, et al. Long-term effect of angiotensin-converting enzyme inhibitor in volume overloaded heart during growth: a controlled pilot study. J Am Coll Cardiol 2000; 36:270–5.

[158] Kouatli AA, Garcia JA, Zellers TM, et al. Enalapril does not enhance exercise capacity in patients after Fontan procedure. Circulation 1997;96:1507–12.

[159] Heragu N, Mahony L. Is captopril useful in decreasing pleural drainage in children after modified Fontan operation? Am J Cardiol 1999;84:1109–12.

[160] Hechter SJ, Fredriksen PM, Liu P, et al. Angiotensin-converting enzyme inhibitors in adults after the Mustard procedure. Am J Cardiol 2001;87:660–3.

[161] Buchhorn R, Hulpke-Wette M, Hilgers R, et al. Propranolol treatment of congestive heart failure in infants with congenital heart disease: The CHF-PRO-INFANT Trial. Int J Cardiol 2001;79:167–73.

[162] Buchhorn R, Bartmus D, Siekmeyer W, et al. Beta-blocker therapy of severe congestive heart failure in infants with left to right shunting. Am J Cardiol 1998;81:1366–8.

[163] Buchhorn R, Ross RD, Hulpke-Wette M, et al. Effectiveness of low dose captopril versus propranolol therapy in infants with severe congestive failure due to left-to-right shunts. Int J Cardiol 2000;76:227–33.

[164] Buchhorn R, Hulpke-Wette M, Ruschewski W, et al. Effects of therapeutic beta blockade on myocardial function and cardiac remodeling in congenital cardiac disease. Cardiol Young 2003;13(1):36–43.

[165] Fernandes SM, Newburger JW, Lang P, et al. Usefulness of epoprostenol therapy in the severely ill adolescent/adults with Eisenmenger physiology. Am J Cardiol 2003;91:632–5.

[166] Galiè N, Ghofrani HA, Torbicki A, et al. Sildenafil citrate therapy for pulmonary arterial hypertension. N Engl J Med 2005;353:2148–57.

[167] Mehta P, Simpson L, Lee E, et al. Endothelin-receptor antagonists improve exercise tolerance and oxygen saturations in adults with the Eisenmenger syndrome [abstract]. Circulation 2005;112:II-680.

[168] Apostolopoulou SC, Manginas A, Cokkinos DV, et al. Long-term clinical, exercise and hemodynamic effect of the endothelin antagonist bosentan in patients with pulmonary arterial hypertension related to congenital heart disease [abstract]. Circulation 2005;112:II-564.

[169] Gatzoulis MA, Rogers P, Li W, et al. Safety and tolerability of bosentan in adults with Eisenmenger physiology. Int J Cardiol 2005;98:147–51.

[170] Schulze-Neick I, Gilbert N, Ewert R, et al. Adult patients with congenital heart disease and pulmonary arterial hypertension: first open prospective multi-center study on bosentan therapy. Am Heart J 2005;150:716.

[171] Galie N, Beghetti M, Gatzoulis M, et al. BREATHE-5: Bosentan improves hemodynamics and exercise capacity in the first randomized placebo controlled trial in Eisenmenger physiology [abstract]. Chest 2005;128:496S.

[172] Piepoli MF, Davos C, Francis DP, et al. ExTraMATCH Collaborative. Exercise training meta-analysis of trials in patients with chronic heart failure (ExTraMATCH). BMJ 2004;328(7433):189.

[173] Therrien J, Fredriksen P, Walker M, et al. A pilot study of exercise training in adult patients with repaired tetralogy of Fallot. Can J Cardiol 2003;19:685–9.

[174] Thaulow E, Fredriksen PM. Exercise and training in adults with congenital heart disease. Int J Cardiol 2004;97(Suppl 1):35–8.

[175] Graham TP Jr, Driscoll DJ, Gersony WM, et al. Task Force 2: congenital heart disease. J Am Coll Cardiol 2005;45(8):1326–33.

[176] Deanfield J, Thaulow E, Warnes C, et al. Management of grown up congenital heart disease. Eur Heart J 2003;24(11):1035–84.

[177] Bolger AP, Coats AJ, Gatzoulis MA. Congenital heart disease: the original heart failure syndrome. Eur Heart J 2003;24(10):970–6.

ELSEVIER
SAUNDERS

CARDIOLOGY
CLINICS

Cardiol Clin 24 (2006) 661–667

# Index

*Note:* Page numbers of article titles are in **boldface** type.

## A

ACC/AHA. See *American College of Cardiology/ American Heart Association (ACC/AHA).*

ACHA. See *Adult Congenital Heart Association (ACHA).*

ACHD. See *Adult congenital heart disease (ACHD).*

Adherence, psychologist's role in ACHD for, 612

Adult Congenital Heart Association (ACHA), 515, 517, 518, 520

Adult congenital heart disease (ACHD)
anesthesiologist's role in, **571–585**
arrhythmias-related, 578–579
cardiac surgery–related, 579–583
ASDs, 580
atrioventricular septal defects, 580
congenitally corrected transposition of great arteries, 582
Ebstein's anomaly, 581
Fontan procedure, 582–583
Glenn procedure, 582–583
PDA, 580
tetralogy of Fallot, 580–581
transposition of great arteries
with Mustard or Senning procedure, 581
with pulmonary stenosis and Rastelli procedure, 582–583
ventricular septal defects, 580
cardioversions, 578–579
diagnostic and interventional services, 578
hypoxemia and shunting–related, 572–573
labor and delivery–related, 579
noncardiac surgery–related, 575–578
described, 575–576
laparoscopic procedures, 577
one-lung ventilation, 577
patient positioning, 576–577
shared airway, 577–578
patient preparation, 573
perioperative TEE, 579

pharmacologic agents–related, 573–575
preoperative assessment, 571–572
regional anesthesia, 575
respiratory issues–related, 572
baroreflex in, 651–652
cardiac catheterization in, **531–556**
aortic valve angiography, 543–544
bidirectional cavopulmonary connection, 546
branch pulmonary artery stenosis, 547
catheter selection for, 532
chamber angiography in, 540–543
changing indications for, 547–552
coarctation of aorta–related, 543
coronary arteriography in, 539–540
cross-sectional imaging and, 550–551
echocardiography and, 549–550
equipment for, 532–536
atrial septic devices, 534–535
balloons, 533–534
catheters, 532, 533
coils, 534
embolization, 534
endovascular stents, 535–536
guide wires, 533
sheaths, 533
ventricular septal devices, 534–535
flows and shunts in, 536–539
future role of, 555
interventions in, 552–555
Mustard baffle, 544–545
planning of, 531–532
problems associated with, 532
pulmonary valve stenosis and tetralogy of Fallot, 546–547
role of, 551–552
secundum ASD and fenestrated Fontan, 545–546
ventricular septal defect–related, 543
chemoreflex sensitivity in, 651–652
exercise intolerance in, **641–660**
assessment of, 641–643
described, 643–646

doi:10.1016/S0733-8651(06)00079-8

Congenital heart disease (CHD)
  complex, young adult with, transition and
    transfer from pediatric to adult care of,
    **619–629.** See also *Transfer; Transition.*
  adult provider services in, 627
  coordinated transfer process, 627–628
  transfer of care obstacles, 625–626
  transition elements, 620, 622–625. See also
    *Transition, elements of.*
  transition models, 621
  transition process goals, 621
  hematologic considerations in,
    anesthesiologist's role in, 573
  pathophysiology of, 572–573
  patient's perspective on, 525–526
  pregnancy and. See also *Pregnancy.*
    risk factors for, 589–593
      fetal risk, 590–592
      for early parental loss or disability, 593
      maternal risk, 589–592
      recurrence of CHD in offspring, 592–593
    team approach to, **587–605**
      contraception-related, 594–595
      frequently asked questions related to,
        602–603
      high-risk labor and delivery team, 602
      high-risk pregnancy team, 601–602
      labor and delivery–related, 598–600
      patient care–related, 593–600
      pediatric reproductive issues team, 601
      prenatal care–related, 595–598
      prepregnancy care and
        counseling–related, 593–594
      termination issues–related, 595
  prevalence of, 587

Contraception, CHD in pregnancy and, 594–595

Coronary arteriography, in cardiac
  catheterization in ACHD, 539–540

Counseling, prepregnancy, for CHD in
  pregnancy, 593–594

Cross-sectional echocardiography, in pulmonary
  incompetence assessment, 635–637

Cross-sectional imaging, in ACHD, 550–551

Cyanosis, exercise effects of, 649–650

Cytokine(s), activation of, exercise and, 651

**D**

Delivery, labor and, CHD during pregnancy and,
  598–600
  anesthesiologist's role in, 579

Developmental/neurocognitive issues, ACHD
  and, psychologist's role in, 612

Disability(ies), invisible, ACHD-related, patient's
  perspective on, 522

Down syndrome, 560, 561–562

Drug(s), for CHD, anesthesiologist's role in,
  573–575

**E**

Ebstein's anomaly, surgery for, anesthesiologist's
  role in, 581

Echocardiography
  cross-sectional, in pulmonary incompetence
    assessment, 635–637
  in ACHD, 549–550
  transesophageal, perioperative, in adults with
    ACHD, anesthesiologist's role in, 579

Education
  ACHD-related, psychologist's role in, 614–615
  patient-physician, ACHD-related, 518–521

Eisenmenger disease, exercise and,
  649–650

Embolization equipment, for cardiac
  catheterization in ACHD, 534

Endothelial system, dysfunction of, exercise and,
  650

Endovascular stents, for cardiac catheterization in
  ACHD, 535–536

Erythrocytosis, secondary, exercise and, 650

Euro Heart Survey, 643

European Task Force, 610

Exercise. See also *Adult congenital heart disease
  (ACHD), exercise intolerance in.*
  anemia and, 650
  arrhythmias and, 648
  chronotropic incompetence and, 648
  components of, 646–649
  cyanosis and, 649–650
  cytokine activation due to, 651
  Eisenmenger disease and, 649–650
  endothelial dysfunction due to, 650
  heart in, 647–649
  medications and, 649
  myocardial perfusion abnormalities and,
    648–649
  pacing and, 648
  pericardial disease and, 649